The Bell Lap

Stories for Compassionate Nursing Care

Muriel A. Murch

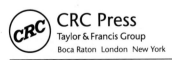

CRC Press
Taylor & Francis Group
Boca Raton London New York

CRC Press is an imprint of the
Taylor & Francis Group, an **informa** business

CRC Press
Taylor & Francis Group
6000 Broken Sound Parkway NW, Suite 300
Boca Raton, FL 33487-2742

Printed on acid-free paper
Version Date: 20160113

International Standard Book Number-13: 978-1-78523-160-5 (Paperback)

Visit the Taylor & Francis Web site at
http://www.taylorandfrancis.com

and the CRC Press Web site at
http://www.crcpress.com

Contents

Acknowledgments   v
Advance Praise for The Bell Lap   vii

Prologue   1
A Drop of Blood   7
The Brigadier, His Buggy and the Butterfly   13
Mr. Tims' Morning   27
It Says Love   33
Morning Coffee   39
The Museum Visit   41
Spring Fever   53
Phone Calls   61
The Waiting Room   71
The Vigil   81
Doctor Patel Comes to Tea   89
The Visitor   99
The Dentist   107
The Letter M   115
Epilogue: A True Story   139

Nursing Notes for The Bell Lap   145
References   151
Index   153
About the Author   155

bell lap

n.

The final lap of a race,
as at a track meet,
signaled by the ringing of a bell
as the leader begins the lap.

Acknowledgments

Throughout our busy nursing lives the writing seed germinates slowly. We snatch moments of quiet time to pull a pen from our pockets and put it to a scrap of paper. Eventually a journal may give way to the notebook and the notebook to produce pages of poetry, memoir or prose, for our muse shows up in different guises.

It is with the help and encouragement of like-minded nurse-writers that I have found my place beside them, and I am forever grateful to the ongoing sisterhood of nurse-writers and physicians who also walk and write in this, our landscape.

Most importantly of all have been the duo of nurse-writers Cortney Davis and Judy Schaefer who edited the writing of nurse-writers from throughout the Western world in their two anthologies, *Between the Heartbeats: Poetry and Prose by Nurses* (1995) and *Intensive Care: More Poetry and Prose by Nurses* (2003). Both anthologies were published by University of Iowa Press.

From these two anthologies have come numerous chapbooks of poetry, memoir and novels written by nurses about nursing and midwifery. Medicine and nursing continue to be a bond that unites us as writers. A huge thank you to Katrina Hulme-Cross who guided me through the publishing process at Radcliffe Publishing and then led me into the safe hands of Naomi Wilkinson when Taylor & Francis took over Radcliffe Publishing.

The following friends, teachers, and writers have all supported, encouraged, and guided this collection of stories. They have corrected and suggested ways that this story could be told this way, or that. Surely mistakes both medical and literary will remain, and those I claim with apologies. Thank you all.

Dorothy Alsup, Melinda Angellini-Hurl, Hal and Barbara Barwood,

Acknowledgments

Mo and Joe Blumenthal MD, Aneta Brown, Ellie Coppola, Sayantani DasGupta MD, Cortney Davis RN, MA, Linda DeLibero, Walter Donahue, Kate Douglas-Henry, Priscilla Ebersole RN, PhD, FAAN, Vibeke Gadd, Megan Gould, Pete Horner, Janet MacIntosh, Beatrice Murch, Walter Murch, Participants of the Sarah Lawrence Medical Writing groups of 2006, Gail Reitano, Janet Robbins, Judy Schaefer and Susan Stone.

The following stories were first published with the rights returned thereafter. I am grateful to these collections and journals.

- *Mr. Tims' Morning* was first published in *Intensive Care: More Poetry and Prose by Nurses*, University of Iowa Press, 2003.
- *The Brigadier, His Buggy and the Butterfly* received a prize from *Lumina Journal*, Sarah Lawrence College, 2007.
- *Doctor Patel Comes to Tea* was first published in *Stories of Illness and Healing: Women Write Their Bodies*, Kent University Press, 2007.
- *A Drop of Blood* was first published by *24/7/365: The International Journal of Healthcare & Humanities*, Volume Three Number Three Spring 2009 and Volume Five Number Five Summer/Fall 2010.
- *Spring Fever* was first published by *24/7/365: The International Journal of Healthcare & Humanities*, Volume Six Number Six Fall/Winter 2011.

A word about names . . .

Though this is a work of fiction I confess that all characters are born from memory and imagination, jumping into the text and making it their own. It can just take an action, a glance, a gesture that gives them birth and a new life.

And for me the truth is that I love the names I know and grew up with. They are comforting to me. They go into a sort of proverbial hat from where I pluck them out. But there are three names I have left in place. In the Prologue, with kind permission from his sister, Graham remains Graham. Sister Boisher was indeed my Sister Tutor. The ward names in *Mr. Tims' Morning* are the ward names I, and others like me, knew and loved as student and staff nurses. In the Epilogue there was no way I could improve on the name Bianca Leonardi.

Advance Praise for
The Bell Lap

Muriel Murch in *The Bell Lap* has explored, with great insight, the multiple lessons of living and dying. With the soul of a poet she delves beyond the surface issues of each caregiving event encountered. She explores beyond visible and concrete experience. In these contributions she has laid the ground for caregivers to reach beyond the confines of the settings of illness, whether home, hospital, long term care, or residential and become an active and involved participant in the world of the other, recognizing that there is no "other." From youth through old age we need wisdom to comprehend this. Reaching beyond the visible to encounter the feelings of family or significant others, and the influence of surroundings. This background is particularly pertinent for the education and development of medical and nursing professionals in this present era of health and illness care when so much has become mechanical and dehumanized. My particular favorites among these stories are: *Mr. Tims' Morning*, *The Waiting Room*, and *Doctor Patel Comes to Tea*. I believe *The Bell Lap* will provide a foundation for compassionate care.

Dr. Priscilla Ebersole PhD, RN, FAAN
Geriatric Nursing Pioneer
Author of *Toward Healthy Aging: Human Needs and Nursing Response*
Geriatric Nursing: Growth of a Specialty

I love these stories! And if you love learning about people from finely tuned fiction, you, too, will love them. And these are stories, true to the marrow, concise and brief, written by a clinician with obvious expertise in the machinations of body and mind—and with obvious comfort in bouts with the spirit. The nuance and descriptive detail of illness and suffering are clinically sound and emotionally poignant.

Nurse Murch knows that each patient has a narrative, a story, of consequence and mystery. Writer Murch turns these narratives end over end like so much evidence that lays out the story of the individual human being, whether patient or professional caregiver. We want to follow the evidence and the timeline and find who and what is at fault. The wordsmithing takes us to the vulnerable edge and we see that there was no crime. There never was, just human beings learning to live and learning to die.

From *Mr. Tims' Morning*, as a nurse myself, I especially like the simplicity of the nurse's words, actions, and plans. In a few words Murch has shown the artfulness of the nurse. I am grateful for this evidence of humanity.

"'Do you need anything?' She asked the question softly, almost vaguely in a manner that allowed him to be slow in his reply. If he chose pain he could receive an opiate. If he chose loneliness she might stay."

In clinical terms nursing and medical students, as well as the general public, will find a new way of understanding complex clinical conditions. *The Bell Lap* will become required reading in healthcare curriculums. In literary terms the reader will find mystery and wordsmithing not unlike O. Henry and atmosphere not unlike Hitchcock. Murch's linguistic clarity and verbal ballet, in itself, is an achievement of a most artful order.

Judy Schaefer, RN, MA
Member, The Kienle Center, College of Medicine, Penn State
  University
Author of *Between the Heartbeats: Poetry and Prose by Nurses*
Wild Onion Nurse
The Poetry of Nursing
Poetry co-editor, *Pulse*, www.pulsevoices.org

With a nurse's careful attention to detail, language and a woman's heart, Murch pulls back the curtain surrounding our hairless, naked, blank-faced bodies and those who stand with us or flee from the house in its decline. Under her umbrella of truth and tenderness, these stories show us how we gather ourselves against the elements, become altered, and go forth carrying our secrets. Murch's voice reassures as our pupils widen and jaws drop. Her eye for the body is a hawk's. She knits her stories of ache and wonder, a geography of relationships where there's no equation to balance, no way to see our ending. To live means we will be reshaped, Murch's stories say over and over, and even if it burns our tongue, love is the tea we share.

Jeanne Bryner, RN, BA, CEN (rtd)
Author of *Tenderly Lift Me: Nurses Honored, Celebrated and Remembered*
Smoke: Poems
Foxglove Canyon

⚜

I loved reading Muriel Murch's *The Bell Lap*. Murch, a registered nurse, writes with the sensitivity, intuition, and attention to nuance that informs her professional caregiving. Each story in this collection is unique, a country unto itself, with characters drawn so clearly and so fully they become not only *known* but *cared about*. I admire Murch's ability to spin tales that not only range the globe but also examine the gamut of human experience: the sweet love, unlike any other, that might develop between patient and nurse; how age encroaches, both challenging and enriching us; how the smallest detail—the blue ceramic coffee pot in the story *Morning Coffee*—becomes a metaphor for what we accept as "normal" until our routines are interrupted by a chronic illness that flares up, then returns us to the mundane where everything is suddenly changed. Like the best British detective, Murch offers us suspense; like the most tender mother she offers us solace; like the excellent author she is, she gives us stories that hold our interest, that inform and afflict us, that are wrought with craft and infused with unforgettable men and women in unforgettable situations. She is also master of the perfect ending. Her stories are never artificially tidied up, but like the bell that signals the bell lap, the one that comes before the final sprint to the end, she allows us, her readers, to deduce what that final journey might entail, how life will end or go on.

But she does not abandon us to face this mystery alone. Murch leaves us always wiser, more aware of the wonder of the human condition, and with more gratitude for every lived moment than we were before we entered "The Bell Lap."

Cortney Davis RN, MA
Author of *Between the Heartbeats: Poetry and Prose by Nurses*
When the Nurse Becomes a Patient: A Story in Words and Images

This collection of wonderful short stories will attract a wide readership. While they mostly deal with medical events, the stories are really about how ordinary people handle life's setbacks. The style is deceptively simple and successfully hides the skilled craftsmanship that keeps the readers' attention from the beginning to the end of each story. Realistic details and fine touches outlining the characters' personalities and reactions allow the reader to participate intimately in their lives. Some of the stories have a melancholic tone, but they are devoid of any hint of sentimentality, another testimony to the author's outstanding literary skills. The most appealing feature of these stories is the irrepressible, life affirming spirit that animates them, that shows people "carrying on" no matter what happens to them.

Anne-Marie Feenberg-Dibon, PhD
Professor, Department of Humanities, Simon Fraser University,
 Vancouver, Canada
Translator of *Malfeasance: Appropriation Through Pollution* by Michel
 Serres

These are stories about intricate caring.
Heartfelt and moving and important.

Michael Ondaatje
Author of *Running in the Family*

The English Patient
The Cat's Table

⁂

Those of us who care for each other can draw comfort and knowledge from Murch's fine stories in *The Bell Lap*. One of my favorites, *The Museum Visit*, tells of the courage it takes to travel out and return to the life we cannot change. A wonderful read for those caring for families and pondering what life has in store for them and all of us.

Eleanor Coppola
Filmmaker, artist and writer
Author of *Notes on a Life*

⁂

We are vain about our bodies. We regard them with passion or despair. And we feel that emotional excess whenever "professionals" study us—doctors, nurses, funerary artists. No need to go that far, perhaps, but the body has its facts that are often beyond deception, or cure. So it's no surprise that medical training and experience are on the way to literary insight. Doctors see many patients, and they know the rules of the game, but somehow it is their oath to look at bodies with as much kindness as honesty. That task is at the heart of Muriel Murch's inspired collection of stories, notes and observations. So this book introduces us to a nurse with a body of her own and a note-taker who is a real writer.

David Thomson
Writer, Film Critic, Historian
Author of *The New Biographical Dictionary of Film*
Moments that Made the Movies

Prologue

FINDING A KINDRED SPIRIT is a gift from the angels. Geography or work may keep you distant but you are always close. You instinctively know that together you face the world looking through the same lens of compassion, understanding and acceptance.

Graham was such a gift. When he came to our city his work encircled the world our family inhabited. We met, not often, but frequently enough, and it was not long before we consciously looked for each other at the film screenings, lectures and awards ceremonies that Graham organized in his role as director of the San Francisco Film Society. Today's Bay Area Film Community is close knit, with more than a forty-year-long history. The jostlings, squabbles, and ownerships of those scrappy young artists have mellowed with the years and given way to mutual admiration for the energy and courage it takes to offer your soul's work to the world. Graham could gently shepherd us all to show up at events in support of one another.

"Oh you are here, it will be all right then," was the message Graham and I took from the reassuring presence of each other. A wave, a twinkling smile, a quick, "How are you doing?" "Fine, and you?" was the most we managed at these times, but they sufficed. We both believed we would, at the end of one such evening, finally sit down with a well-earned glass of wine. Graham would loosen whatever bound him. I would kick off my shoes, and we would laughingly cement the connection we shared.

Then Graham became ill; suddenly, ferociously, and terminally ill. When I heard of his illness, and that he had resigned from his position, I wrote to him and said,

Well bother and bother again . . .

Don't know what sort of shape or frame of mind you are in and if you are receiving visitors. This old nurse doesn't mind illness and sometimes comes

to the city bearing greengage plums or other farm treats. It would be great to see you but if you would rather not I do understand.

He wrote back immediately,

Bother, you say, and bother again. That must be a nurse's restraint kicking in. I tend toward the more purple invective, but in truth it doesn't seem to help any more than gentle displeasure. I'm stuck with this for the duration, I'm sorry to say, and can influence only what that duration might be, and then only marginally, I expect. . . .

So, I find myself waking up each morning with two somewhat but not entirely compatible tasks: living longer and dying well. A lot of the time they overlap, but not always. Encouragement like yours and the extraordinary friends I have make it that much easier to press on and let the devil take the hindmost—forgetting as often as I can that it is probably me who IS the hindmost. Ha ha! . . .

It's funny that you should say I make you feel safe since you have exactly that effect on me, especially in the half-chaotic settings in which we meet. . . .

Good to find kin and even better to find spirit . . .

To that end, yes, please, come over anytime, with or without food. Just bring yourself and we'll drink tea and have a good chat.

So it was arranged. I drove to the city, parked, entered his apartment building and rode the elevator up to the third floor. Graham poked his shiny bald head, that now looked shockingly heavy and way too big for his shrunken frame, out of his doorway.

Grinning his mischievous grin he beckoned me in. He made a cup of tea for me and gave himself a quick injection of something stronger before we sat down for the catch-up chat that we had both waited too long for.

We came from different parts of the U.K., Graham from the North, I from the South, and different social backgrounds, but there were no core beliefs or values we did not share. After an hour, time, energy, and comfort ran out for Graham, and we said our goodbyes. We planned another meeting when he and his girlfriend, Diana, returned from a week's holiday in Italy. But the next week he wrote again. They were not going to Italy. His doctor had advised he stay at home—and rest.

"I guess I have entered The Bell Lap." Graham wrote. He died two weeks later.

While I write, the greengage plums are ripening on the tree again.

Another friend has entered his *Bell Lap*. As a friend and a nurse, I will travel part of that journey with him and his family, knowing, as I do, something of the nature of the disease that is claiming him.

～○※～

During the final summer of my school days, the one that brings the understanding that this is childhood's twilight with the dawn of adulthood still far away, I spent the weekday afternoons at our local cottage hospital. I would walk from home, turning left along Elvetham Road and left again up Stockton Avenue and into the hospital driveway. Working as what in America would be called a Candy Striper, I would tidy beds, help with flower arranging, always a big job in those days before flowers arrived prearranged, and serve tea. Sometimes, after I had put away the tea trolley and straightened the last of the beds, an old friend of my parents would collect me and take me with him to visit patients at home. Doctor Riley was a tall distinguished-looking man who made many housewives' hearts flutter. But I wasn't sure what to make of him or these late afternoon car rides and visits to people's homes that I would never normally enter. He was still cresting the prime of his career. Not yet, I think, aware that the tide of his life too would ebb and retreat. Doctor Riley was a fine physician in the old school at a time when the art of medicine rode in tandem with the science. On these afternoon trips he began to teach me that the body can, at times, heal itself with a little encouragement and confidence and that when it could not, when disease meandered slowly or raced furiously through a body, neither he nor his colleagues were always able to change its course.

One afternoon we drove to a row of cottages and knocked on the door of Number Fourteen. The cottage smelt musty, with that closed-in, old-people-who-want-to-stay-warm smell. If my memory is correct, an old woman was fading into congestive heart failure. There Dorothy sat, breathless, in her chair downstairs. "It's too much to go up to bed, Doctor." Albert, her husband, retired from a life shoveling coal on the railway, hovered, shuffling between the living room and the kitchen, and making anyone he could a strong cup of tea. Dorothy, overflowing from the stuffed, and maybe sodden, chair waved him away with one hand as she struggled to talk to Doctor Riley who stood and then quietly sat beside her. He listened intently, receiving her as she breathlessly told him how she felt, how her husband was worn down with the work of caring for her. Unspoken between them lay her question, how long would Albert have to carry on? Eventually we said our goodbyes and left, ducking our heads under the low cottage door frame. But the day's lesson was not over.

As we drove back along Elvetham Road, we passed a man I recognized slightly. He was walking, bowed over a cane and with a concentrated, lopsided smile that, combined with the cane-assisted walk, gave him a crazed look as he slowly made his way along the pavement.

"What do you think is wrong with Mr. Nieto?" asked Doctor Riley. I had no idea. Whenever I saw Mr. Nieto I shied away from him. His strange walk, smile and strange name intimidated and scared me as all things that are odd do to teenagers. Slowly Doctor Riley began to explain multiple sclerosis, to the depth of understanding that science had reached in the early 1960s.

Three years later, while I was a student nurse and rotating through Edward, the male neurological ward, Mr. Nieto became my patient. He still had the same crooked, cheerful smile while he lay in bed. A urinary catheter was in place and drained his cloudy waste into a bag not too discreetly tucked under the covers. He had been admitted with pneumonia and, with his reduced lung capacity, was very ill. I remember that I was no longer afraid of his strangeness, and I would like to think that it was remembering how he had walked down Elvetham Road years ago that helped me be a better nurse to him and others.

Mr. Nieto has long shuffled away to a greater comfort than he found on this earth. But what remains is the gift that Doctor Riley gave me: to look at people, to see or imagine their lives as well as the age and illness that they carry. That seeing is a gift I have treasured since I first realized that the people I nursed were loved and cared for by others, while they suffered the changes in body and mind that are disease.

When Graham gave me the title of this collection, he also gave me much to think about. The stories that make up *The Bell Lap* have been created out of memories, imaginings and love.

Doctor Clark-Kennedy wrote *Medicine in its Human Setting* (Faber and Faber, London, 1954/61) while he was a teaching physician at The London

Hospital in England and Doctor Riley was a young intern. Doctor Riley followed Clark-Kennedy on his rounds, tended his patients and learned his lessons, of people, patients and their diseases. It was Sister Tutor Boisher, a contemporary of Doctor Riley's, who handed this slim volume to me. It is a book I love, and it has stayed close by my side, traveling from home to home since 1962. It is the seed that germinated *The Bell Lap*.

These stories are not about death, though death is present in some, but about the advancement of age and illness and the changes that come to us in this life. The stories ask: at what point in life's journey do each of us enter our *Bell Lap*? How does it happen? Do we recognize it when it does happen? How do we face to it? Or in Graham's own words how do we face the:

> two somewhat but not entirely compatible tasks: living longer and dying well.

M.A.M., 2015

A Drop of Blood

AS HE STEPS OUT of the shower he notices the drop of blood on the white marble bathroom floor. Tony Beal and his wife Sarah are in Rome on one of the working trips that double for them as a vacation. Sarah has long ago given up on real holidays. These working trips come their way frequently as Tony's reputation as a speaker has grown to match his one as a gifted neurosurgeon.

This Rome conference is an international gathering of neurosurgeons. Though most of the surgeons know of each other by reputation, referral and their published monographs, these conference gatherings are an opportunity to travel and mingle safely in like-minded company. A neurosurgeon, perhaps more than any other physician, prefers not to be surprised by the people he meets. Few neurosurgeons are women. Women have the dexterity and finesse for the surgery but this brotherhood still doubts their ability to carry the emotional or physical weight needed to pull hard on a cracked skull.

Now that their two children are through college, married and with families of their own, Sarah enjoys joining Tony at the conferences. As a younger woman she was withdrawn. While engaging in her children's school activities she managed to overcome some of her shyness but she never became really comfortable at the functions Tony asked her to share with him then. She has become lonely at home and, in her heart, admits to pangs of jealousy for Tony's freedom and ability to enjoy himself, with or without her, when he is away. But she has grown bolder with age and now she too enjoys visiting other cities, meeting some of the other wives, who have also been as lonely as she once was. Much of the time she spends discovering her own mind, her own thoughts, ones that she didn't know she possessed. She also sleeps recovering from a deep fatigue, unknowing of its source, that also surprises her. Living and working beside Tony has been like working a waitress's split shift, though without the split break in between.

She begins this trip to Rome by walking aimlessly, until Tony is ready to join her. Later they walk together through parks, wander into museums, attend concerts, and browse other cultural interests. Tony's knowledge of history and music make these times more enjoyable. She knows he loves telling her things. Teaching is second nature to him as it is to any man who passionately loves his chosen work.

Tony is an exemplary neurosurgeon. Residents chosen to rotate by his side go on to excel in their own practices. To have scrubbed beside Tony Beal in the big New York teaching hospital would, unless one cracked, set up a young surgeon for a successful practice.

But on this, the second morning of their week-long stay in Rome, Tony was not thinking of his successes as he stepped out of the shower onto the warm bathroom floor of their elegant hotel. There was blood on the floor. He was always watchful. Blood on the floor was something he knew about. On entering a fresh surgical suite his eyes would take in the whole room, the gleaming clean steel, the bright lights, the trays of equipment laid out ready for his use, the crisp scrub uniforms of the surgical team, nurses, technicians, the anesthesiologist already attached to and caring for the patient—and the spotlessly clean surgical floor. The staff stood in a regimented order for his inspection and approval before he'd approach the patient. Like an old sea-captain he needed to know everything was in its place and as it should be before setting sail into the skull and mind of a fellow human being. Once he was satisfied, he would then step forward, his registrars and interns following behind him as in a choral wave.

But this morning when he stepped out of the shower he saw the spot of blood. It was not a big spot. It was not old, dark, and dry. As he looked around, he saw two new splotches. They were small, seeming to spread like a tiny leaf but one without the veined pattern of the autumnal leaves he knew. Had Sarah nicked her ankle while shaving her legs? Sometimes that happened when she used a fresh razor at home. Had he nicked himself? He leaned forward towards the mirror and absentmindedly reached out for a towel and rubbed his cheeks, though he hadn't shaved yet that morning. The towel in his hand absorbed the water from his face but came away clean.

"Sarah, there's blood on the bathroom floor." He called to her through the half-open door to the bedroom. Sarah was sitting on the bed, still wearing the thick hotel robe that she loved to lounge in during these holiday interludes.

"Hum," she replied.

"Have you cut yourself?" Tony asked, neither academically nor kindly, not yet on the scent of a trail, but searching, as if for the answer to a crossword puzzle, for the clue to the blood on the floor.

"No, I haven't," Sarah replied absentmindedly. But she too began to think about the blood.

Tony shaved, cleaned his teeth with the disciplined thoroughness he used for all his morning ablutions and looked at himself again in the mirror. He held his head up high, searching for stray soap or whiskers whose remnants would make him seem old and forgetful. He has always held an impatience, a slight sneer for those of his colleagues who didn't keep up their appearances. There was nothing wrong with his face, he thought, it was still handsome. He combed his hair carefully. He still had a good head of hair, a little thin at the back maybe but he could hardly see that from the front and was only reminded of this slight to his vanity as he passed a comb over his head. He gave a little nod to the mirror and himself as he finally shook the towel free of his shoulders, dropping it to the floor before striding into the bedroom. The towel lay crumpled where he left it and the blood, which had softened with the moisture and warmth of his shower, now started to solidify again as the temperature and humidity in the bathroom began to fall.

"Are you finished?" Sarah looked up at her husband and smiled.

"Yes. It's all yours my dear." Tony's tone was affectionate. The memory of the blood receded. He was looking at his wife of thirty-five years. Sexual passion had always ebbed and flowed through their long marriage and now, with rest, the familiarity of desire began to rise in him. Loving trust had overcome the fear that turbulent years of his early successes in their marriage had brought. They recognized each other as the best friend they each had, and like the friends they each made over the years they loved each other despite their faults and frailties. They knew each other's moods, knew the signals of desire and need, to be close or to be left alone.

Sarah got up from the bed, went to the bathroom and closed the door.

She sat down on the wide marble edge of the bathtub and looked at the floor. She smiled. She wondered what Tony had been talking about. It never occurred to Tony to clean up, to wipe away the blood from the floor with his used towel. She picked up the used towel he had dropped on the floor. She looked down and then she saw them, two spots of blood, small, dried and dark. Not much she thought, not really fresh either, but where did they come from? She ran her hands over her calves and looked down at her ankles. There were no nicks or red slashes showing. The angle of the razor had been true. So where had the blood come from?

Sarah picked up the wet towel again. She held it up, looking for signs of blood. There were none. She thought about Tony, mentally checking over his body with the mind of a wife and mother who had learnt enough to watch for the physical signs of disease in the bodies of those she loved. Tony's body was good, trim though not tight. A few loose ripples rather than rolls about his midriff. His buttocks were no longer round and firm, though they could and did tighten well, she thought with a smile. His legs, the last to go, as her grandmother had told her, were still slim and fine. They would be considered stringy if his meat was on the butcher's block. She shook herself. Where did that housewifery thought come from? Blood she thought, that's where. Her shoulders sank down as her spine curved, lacking the strength to hold her upright for the moment. Where did the blood come from? She knew it was not from her body. There were no telltale signs of mucus, or bloodstained tissue. She felt no pain. She checked her feet for cracked soles but from just three days of cosseted care her feet were already smoother than they had been for months.

Together Sarah and Tony finished getting dressed and left the hotel to find an espresso coffee bar outside. Tony had the day free and they decided to spend the morning walking in the Villa Borghese and the afternoon further afield wandering through the Coliseum. The sun was shining, the temperature was not yet too hot. The air was fresh with the promise of autumn into winter. By the time they met their friends Jane and Peter for dinner they were hungry. The evening was filled with relaxed friendship, good conversation, and Italian provincial food. A lovely day ended in an easy evening, they both thought as they walked happily back to the hotel that night.

Their room was fresh and welcoming as a four star hotel should be.

The bed was already turned down and the comforter lay inviting them to sex or sleep. The bathroom was clean with fresh towels and soap. Sarah's cosmetics were laid out neatly on a face cloth. Sarah always smiled looking at the way different hotel maids cared for her most personal implements. They prepared for bed and snuggled down into the gentleness of each other's bodies and sleep. The desire that was rising in both of them had been subdued for the night by a good wine with their dinner.

Tony woke early and from a deep sleep and reached for the soft warmth of Sarah's body. He took her differently now. Sometimes on mornings such as these she made her body welcoming, wetting her fingers in her mouth, moving them across her sex, allowing his entry to the moisture that still lay inside her. She welcomed his body and he responded to her welcome like an old warrior. He was grateful for these mornings when she asked for nothing in return. Later they lay together and dozed before Tony rose, satisfied and proud, to shower in the bathroom. Sarah lay in bed, closing her eyes to doze some more. She woke as Tony leaned over her, dressed, ready to lecture and face the world of his own creation. He carried the confidence of every man successful at copulation. After the door had closed on him Sarah slowly got up, put her feet into the waiting slippers and went to the bathroom. She sat down on the toilet and emptied her bladder before reaching for the robe hanging behind the door. She filled a glass of water and took her morning handful of vitamin pills. Then she sat down on the wide bathtub edge to think about the day ahead of her. What to do? Where to go? As she held the half empty glass of water in her hand she glanced down at the bathroom floor. Yesterday's marks were gone but beside the bath mat, outside of the shower, there was another fresh drop of blood.

The Brigadier, His Buggy and the Butterfly

IT WOULD HAVE BEEN over a year since Colonel Crawly had first diagnosed Brigadier Reginald Armstrong's aortic aneurysm.

"You're lucky we found it sir," the young army lieutenant resident said just before Colonel Crawly, his consultant physician, had returned to the room.

The brigadier snorted at the impertinence, lucky indeed, to find he had a weak heart. How dare the lieutenant imply that the brigadier had a weakness. He had stout-heartedly dismissed the ailments as age encroached through his life like a housing development creeping down to the shores of a tranquil bay. Arthritis and constipation had joined a hernia for himself and failing eyesight for his wife, Sheila. Still there must be something to this heart business; Crawly looked grave when he came into the consulting room.

"Good morning Brigadier. Has my young lieutenant been talking with you this morning?" The question hung in the room addressed to both men.

"Some nonsense about a dicky heart." Armstrong's tone was brusque. He knew these young chaps. They would shout out some problem, click their heels with a "sir," and then watch, hoping you would make a duff of it. Not him by jove; he'd been there, pulled the same tricks himself as a young soldier, hadn't he?

Colonel Crawly sat down in his chair and rested his arms on the desk before he leaned forward and continued, "I've been looking at the tests results from last week and it's a bit serious I'm afraid." It was never *very* serious between army men. A situation could be a *bit* serious or even *rather* serious. "Maybe I should have said *rather*," thought the colonel to himself. "Armstrong can be a thick old bird." He swiveled his chair around and stood holding the X-rays up, checking if he had them the right way around before clipping them onto the lit screen behind him.

"Come and take a look at this." Armstrong got up and moved behind the desk to stand beside Crawly. Together they studied the chest X-rays. Crawly briefed the brigadier as if it was a battlefront map. He pointed out the good areas first.

"Chest cage looks pretty healthy, lungs are clear and strong, top tubing good, here's your heart and the plumbing below." The heart was captured in the black and white negative X-ray slung like an antique oil rig, pausing only for the camera shutter as it sucked blood from the lungs and pumped it back to the body.

"The heart is enlarged a bit. It is not too much of a problem in itself but here is the difficulty." His forefinger, which had been moving across the X-ray in large sweeping movements, stopped at the aorta.

"See this bulge here?" Crawly waited for the brigadier to focus on the spot before continuing. "That is *rather* serious I'm afraid."

They stood together in silence for a full half-minute. The brigadier crossed his arms over his chest and cupped his chin in his right hand. In truth he didn't really grasp what Crawly was talking about.

"How serious?" he eventually asked, knowing that another question would buy him more time.

"It's a weakness," responded Crawly. The brigadier flinched again at that word, "in the wall of the aorta. A bit like a tire before it is going to burst. It could go at any time. Nowadays we can repair them if we can catch them in time. I'll fix up for you to see Major-General Martin. He's a good man, vascular surgeon, we can do it here of course, he comes down, no need to go to London if you don't want to." Giving the brigadier a choice about where to have the surgery would be another way to help move the old boy towards accepting it. Crawly knew that the brigadier was not going to go along easily with this turn to his life. Who would, he thought to himself. He spoke quickly, wanting to get the bad news across without too much discussion.

But the brigadier had always taken bad news on board slowly, much like a dredging barge chugging along old canals loading up with the sludge of overgrown weeds that slowed the waters. His stubbornness had been an asset to him as a desk-bound soldier and his reluctance to make snap decisions had left him time to form alternate, obscure ideas. In those moments of steady methodical thought he had solved knotty logistical problems with seemingly effortless brilliance and gained the respect of both his men and commanders. He felt again a familiar caution about the terrain he was entering, so he paused before asking, "And what would this Martin feller want to do?" He didn't like the idea of someone mucking about with his heart's plumbing.

"Well, it's quite good actually. They can go in and patch it up. Won't last forever of course, but should give you another short innings."

"And what happens if I don't see this chap?" Armstrong asked this question slowly.

"Well," Crawly spoke slower now too. "You've a bit of a time bomb I'm afraid. It could blow at any time, give or take a year, really. Easy for you of course old man, but what about Sheila?"

Reg did not say much to Sheila that day when he returned home after the appointment with Colonel Crawly. He was upset and felt pushed, knowing that the decision was already made for him. He could either carry on and die a coward and selfish husband or, for Sheila's sake as well as his own, go ahead with the surgery. But he didn't like it. No, he didn't like it at all.

⁂

A few days later, Reg returned home early from the golf club where he had gone to play nine holes but had instead found himself staying on the practice putting green. At lunch he announced to Sheila that he had decided to have that operation Crawly was on about. The fifty years of marriage behind them had honed his style. He announced his decision and waited for Sheila to accommodate any problems created by his pronouncement.

As an army couple it was not until their forties that Reg and Sheila bought their first house, in preparation for their retirement. Hartly Mow was a tidy home county's village that, like a lake receiving small country streams, absorbed its complement of retired army commanders and docked them comfortably in the village, the church, and on the old golf course. With Reg's retirement had come increased time together, though in their moments alone each had separate wistful thoughts of what they might have missed in a possibly more intimate family relationship.

Sheila had gone on organizing their lives through the years of retirement and they had managed comfortably. Reg's consultation work had kept him pretty busy. He had faithfully put some savings away along with his army pension and felt he had done well in providing for them. But now came this jolt to his security. He wasn't ready for a brush with the life hereafter and was doubtful that his dutifulness as a church warden had fooled the God that his wife believed in so fervently.

Later that week, Reg returned to the golf club. He walked slowly from his parked car towards the old shed that sat between the parking lot and the practice ground. The shed was now so old and decrepit that it was treasured as quaint. Here he kept his golf buggy, a privilege extended to less than half a dozen of the also old and decrepit senior members. The buggy was dark green and the crustings of mud that lay over the wheel casings gave it an air of appropriate seriousness, an almost military persona, that suited Reg. The sky was overcast and dull. He felt the weight of the rain in the clouds and the oppression of what lay before him. Damn it, he thought, if I don't have the operation people will say I am selfish. Why, Crawly had almost said as much. "What about Sheila?" he had said. Blast it, his trusted seven iron stuck as he tried to take the club from his bag. She can take care of herself, always had, she pretends she needs me but it is a sham, just trying to make up for—suddenly he pressed his lips together for a sadness had risen from his heart to his throat, like a misplaced erection that he still wasn't sure what to do with. Damn. Why should he have to do this, he asked himself, but the question unfolded his answer. It was the same as before the war, a brigadier in the engineering corps, sitting back in the office not really getting into the action. Well, he didn't like getting dug in, he thought angrily, didn't like engagement, never had.

"Good afternoon, sir." Reg turned around slowly, straightening his back a little with the knowledge that he was one of the few members left that was still addressed as sir. Nigel Pearce, a tall man in his forties, had stopped by the open shed door and was smiling in at him.

"What are you up to?" replied Reg crossly. Here it was again, engagement when he didn't want it. Nigel was unfazed by the brigadier, and smiled confidently at the old man.

"Just a few practice balls with my son. Lovely afternoon."

Reg grunted and shoved his truculent seven iron back in the bag and the bag back into his buggy.

"Cheerio then." Nigel smiled again as he turned to leave. Reg continued to glower at his back. He turned back to his bag, surprisingly thinking about Nigel, carrying on, playing with his son. Reg didn't have a son but understood that if he didn't want to stop living then he too must carry on. The brief exchange made Reg realize there was no escape at all. He would have to have the surgery.

Sheila had told her bridge group of course. The ladies were attentive and in complete agreement with Sheila's decision to go ahead with her own needed eye surgery before Reg had his heart operation.

"Otherwise, how am I to take care of him?" Her friends nodded their assent.

So it was arranged. Sheila had one eye done immediately and successfully. Six weeks later she returned for the second eye, and although the surgery was again successful, the recovery was flawed. She felt Reg's agitation and, as ever trying to accommodate him, she did too much too early and developed a spot, floating on her retina. Guilt and fear made Reg angry and snappish with her before it was all over.

⁂

It was the end of June by the time Reg went into hospital for his surgery.

"You've got the heart of a man half your age," the young doctors told him, one by one, as they all filed through his room with their endless admission forms and with only the slightest variance on words. He was gratified by their remarks, although when the doctors had left and Sheila had gone home and the nurses said goodnight to him, he wondered why then, with the heart of a younger man, did he have to be here?

The night sedation did not help him sleep even though the only pills he ever took were the big yellow multivitamin jobs that Sheila pressed on him every day at breakfast. At one o'clock in the morning he was awake and hungry and rang the bell to call the nurse.

"I cannot sleep. I want a glass of warm milk. Please." He added the please as a concession. She was a pretty young thing and he had not seen her before.

"I'm sorry Brigadier Armstrong, it is too late, you cannot have anything more to eat or drink until after your operation." He stared at her glumly. Orders are orders but he still hated taking someone else's. He was hungry and felt peevishly cross. The nurse was young and slightly afraid of the brigadier. She looked again at his chart and came back into the room.

"You can have another sleeping pill if you like."

He snorted, "No thank you. I just want a glass of milk. Then I can go to sleep."

"I'm sorry. Is there anything else I can get you?" The young nurse stood by the door nervously, wanting to go but knowing she must leave him vaguely contented.

"No. Thank you," he replied and, clutching the bed clothes, drew the sheet up to his chest.

"Just ring the bell if you need anything."

Reg spent the rest of the night dozing fitfully until he was woken by his sluggish but insistent bladder at five-thirty in the morning. He sighed and climbed out of the unfamiliar bed like a condemned man accepting the dawning of his execution day.

At seven, Major-General Martin came in looking like a mature gladiator, glistening with early-morning, early middle-aged health.

"Good morning Brigadier. Are you all ready for me this morning?"

"Good morning." Reg realized he had forgotten the man's name and asked, in an effort to bluster, "Are you ready for me—eh?"

"Oh yes. Absolutely. The team is upstairs getting everything together now. We will be giving you some more medication soon. Mrs. Armstrong will be in before you come up, won't she?'

"Here I am." Sheila appeared behind the surgeon wearing the painted bright smile she had perfected over the years hosting for Reg and his guests. She looked neat. Her single-strand pearl necklace lay gently around her neck. She wore a fresh lavender blouse under a gray cardigan and her light tweed skirt and slip-on shoes were smart and comfortable. She was dressed for a long day of waiting.

"Good morning, Doctor. Good morning, dear. How did you sleep?" Sheila's heart's attention for once overtook her good manners.

"Didn't sleep a damn. Nurse wouldn't give me a glass of milk."

Major-General Martin took this as his cue.

"The nurse will be with you shortly and I'll see you both again as soon as you come up. I'll leave him to you Mrs. Armstrong." And he walked briskly out of the room with the firm authority of a busy man.

Reg hardly remembered the nurse coming in and starting the intravenous drip and administering the preoperative medication. Dimly he was conscious of Sheila sitting beside him and holding his hand tenderly before they wheeled him away. Martin was ready for him. The surgery was a good teaching experience for the residents who knew when they entered their rotation with Major-General Martin they would learn from one of the best vascular surgeons in England. The fact that he had chosen to remain and work in the army only enhanced his reputation as a man dedicated to the heart's call of surgery and who had rejected the cup of fame. After opening the chest and exposing the brigadier's steadfastly beating heart, Martin pointed out the aneurysm to the students before continuing to talk and work efficiently through the procedure. After the repair was completed he slipped his fingers underneath the beating heart, cradled it gently and spoke softly.

"Look at it gentlemen. Look at it and wonder." The students were quiet as the surgery ended. The most senior resident assisted with the suturing while Martin reiterated the procedure completed and continued to outline the brigadier's treatment they would be responsible for over the next few days.

The effects of the surgery, age, and medication blended the next two days and nights together. Nightmares eventually gave way to dreams and when Reg finally woke up it was to a slow consciousness of surprise and relief. The doctors came to his bedside, briefly, to effuse at what a success he was. The nurses clucked him along much too quickly for his liking. They got him up and out of bed. Inhalation and physical therapists came to make him breathe and walk, allowing no physical stagnation. Reg had lost more confidence than he realized and his body felt strangely unfamiliar. But the therapists overrode Reg's mental agitation in this rush to recovery. He made good progress and was discharged with no complications. But as he waited in the hospital lobby, sitting in a wheelchair clutching a basket of half-eaten fruit, for Sheila to bring the car to the entrance, he wondered how on earth he was going to manage.

Over the first few days at home Reg moved cautiously around the house and Sheila stayed close by his side. Traveling to and from the hospital and supplying the constant cheerfulness Reg needed had left her sapped of energy by the time he returned home. But by the following Thursday afternoon Sheila was ready to go to the hairdresser. Instead of closing the front door for his departing wife, Reg clicked the latch onto safety and walked across the road to the church. The air was fresh and he felt less tired than he had supposed he would. Maybe he was going to get better, he thought to himself. Returning to the house, he went to the kitchen and opening the freezer found a container of ice cream. He sat down in the sitting room and turned on the television to watch the Scottish open golf championship. It was here that Sheila found him asleep on her return. The television was still on but now blaring out the Telly Tubbies song and an empty ice cream container was on the floor beside his chair.

Three weeks later, Sheila drove Reg back to the doctor's clinic for a check-up. There was a new young registrar who had not had the time to read through the brigadier's notes. He asked old questions as well as new, to which Reg responded in a crusty, military manner. Major-General Martin came in and put his hand out to receive the medical chart from his new registrar.

"Hello again. How have you been feeling?" Martin listened to Reg's reply as he read the new registrar's notes, looking for information and slips to correct the youngster in front of Reg. Nothing like a little instruction to remind the brigadier who was boss here.

"Let's get your shirt off and take a listen to you." When Reg was ready, Martin paused for a still moment admiring his handiwork before bending over and placing the stethoscope down on the folded white flesh of Reg's chest. Really the old boy was amazing. The heartbeat through the stethoscope was steady and strong, the river of blood safely passed by the tight-knit seams. As Martin leaned over the brigadier he wondered how much time he had given him. How much more could he do? There was no fault, no flaw with the surgery or the results, but the heart beat with a precariousness that Martin only could sense. Maybe this awesome responsibility was the legacy he was given from holding this heart literally in his hands.

Reg lay still, looking neither to the right nor the left and certainly not at Martin. Instead he fixed his eyes on the curtains drawn around him in the vicinity of his left foot. Martin listened some more and then straightened up and smiled brightly.

"Very good. Do you mind?" He moved his arm and still holding his stethoscope waved it in the direction of the resident. "I'd like him to have a listen."

Reg nodded his assent but neither man paid any further attention to the young doctor as he too listened to the steadily beating heart.

"So what's the verdict?" Reg asked.

"You're a free man. We'll want to keep an eye on you of course, and check some blood levels every few weeks. Crawly will take care of that from home and make sure that your medication is still on track with the test results. Other than that it is back to normal for you. Do what you feel like and want to do. Can't make you a young man of forty I'm afraid, but some things will be easier than they have in the last year or two."

Reg didn't ask—for how long. Instead he said, "And golf?"

"Absolutely, you have your golf buggy. Take it slow, and stay on the practice grounds at first but then there is no reason why you shouldn't play a few holes when you feel ready. Take Sheila out for a drive on the course. It will do you both good. I'll see you again in six weeks." Martin stood back and turned aside so he would not watch as the young doctor helped the old brigadier sit up and put his shirt back on.

⚜

Two days later, over breakfast on a not too warm and not too sunny day, Reg announced he would go down to the club that morning.

"Would you like me to come with you?" asked Sheila.

"No, thank you," Reg replied carefully, "I'm just going to check over the buggy."

"You'll be back for lunch?" She had perfected the statement, a cross between a question and a command, and he knew enough to listen.

"Oh, a couple of hours should do it." He wanted to reassure her and himself that he would be back. He checked his keys, his rain jacket, put on his cap and went out to the car. He sat in the driver's seat for a full couple of minutes looking at all the dials as if for the first time. Calming himself, he breathed in deeply before turning the key in the ignition and backing slowly out of the driveway and turning onto the road. None of his reflexes were slower, everything moved the same, he could drive. He took the back route along Avenue Road down by the railway line. He looked anew, as if he had returned from a long tour of duty abroad, at the ramblings of the overgrown perennial flowers in what used to be the allotment gardens of the railway cottages. The cottages were no longer lived in by the railway workers, who could not afford to buy them when they had been sold off for profit by the railway companies. The new owners had turned the front flower gardens into carports and the old allotments that had been the bridge from starvation to survival between the two great wars were left fallow. Small apples were beginning to peek through the dark green leaves on an old Bramley apple tree that bent over the wire fence. Wild mullein blossoms swayed in the breeze stirred by the passing cars. On the other side of the road the lush green foliage of the rhododendrons, whose blossoms had long since passed, stood guard over the deep driveways leading up to ever more expensive suburban houses. He drove along slowly, comforted by this familiar road.

Reg arrived at the club safely and parked in a slot close to the shed where he kept his buggy. As he turned the engine off he sat still for a moment, absorbing the familiar scene. A shadow came over his view and he looked up to see Nigel Pearce's blue-sweatered belly blocking his window. Nigel waved and stepped out of the way so that Reg could get out of the car. Reg opened the door and stuck his head out. Surprised at himself, he was glad to see that someone was at the club to welcome him. He had hoped to be missed and now was grateful for the reassurance of a friendly face.

"Well, if it isn't the brigadier. Good to see you back, sir. How are you feeling?" Nigel's cheerfulness used to grate on Reg but not today.

"Well," he must make this last he realized, "not too bad all things considered. Glad to be standing."

"Next you'll be swinging a club I suppose," replied Nigel. Damn the man and his observant optimism thought Reg.

"Thought I would just come down and check over the old buggy."

"The course has dried up a bit since you've been gone; we could do with some rain." Nigel looked up at the sky and the oncoming clouds.

"Won't get much today," Reg said flatly. He had always been able to read the weather but now his body picked up more through the pores of his skin and the arthritis in his joints than his nose or his eyes.

Reg locked his car carefully and put the keys in his trouser pocket. The two men walked together towards the shed which housed the buggies. Nigel lingered while Reg reached back into his trouser pocket for another fistful of keys and separated them through his fingers as he searched by feel for the one that would open the shed. When Nigel saw that Reg had the key, he raised his hand.

"Must be off, sir. Going out for a few holes with Geoffrey. Good to see you." Nigel walked away smiling. That heart operation doesn't seem to have changed the old boy any, he thought.

"You too. Bye." Reg's mind was now on the key to the shed and what he would find inside. He unlocked the shed and opened the wide, wood door, allowing light to shine in like a weak torch onto the four golf carts parked at the back of the shed. Reg was relieved to see his buggy in the gloom, looking exactly as he had left it, like a patient old dog waiting for its master. Ghostly nightmares had left him afraid it would have been moved, taken away, as he knew it would be, when the day came that he failed to return.

He walked over and took the cover off the seat. Slowly he climbed on board and turned the key. The engine coughed, clearing its throat discreetly, before rising to attention and moving the current of electricity through the machine and coming to life. Reg let the brake out, turned the steering wheel, and put his foot on the throttle. Slowly he maneuvered out of the shed and into the parking lot, applying the brake as he pulled up alongside his car. He went back to lock the shed door before taking a handful of clubs and a tube of golf balls from the boot of his car and transferring them onto the back of the buggy. He released the brake once more and slowly drove off to the practice ground. The rubber tires propelled the buggy along the grass like a park donkey stepping happily out in the sunlight, taking the first youngster of the day for a ride. The hum of the machine was quietly in keeping with the lazy birdsong of an early summer morning.

Reg drove to the far edge of the practice ground and parked. He had no plan in his mind but reached for his favorite seven iron that had become dearer to him as his capacity for a few holes had diminished. The balls rolled out of his plastic pipe and into the grass that was on the long side of trim. It was not yet time for the weekly mowing and the grass grew fast here in this shaded corner.

After a couple of reflex practice swings Reg addressed the first of his balls as if he had never been away or ill. In fact he hit about ten balls quite well before he paused. By jove, not bad all things considered, he thought. He stood up for a moment to stretch before readdressing the next group of balls. As so often happens in golf, his new consciousness made him shift his stance just enough that he duffed the next half-dozen balls. Even bringing himself up to refocus, he still did not hit the remaining balls well and by the time he clambered back into his buggy he was hot and cross. Roughly he switched on the ignition, took a firm hold of the steering wheel with one hand and reached for his plastic collection ball tube with the other. He put his foot down fast on the throttle but had forgotten to release the hand brake and the buggy stalled with a hiccup, so he had to turn the ignition on again. He drove towards the first ball lying innocently on the grass. As he bent over low, down went his arm and the plastic pole sucked up the first of the now passive balls. Again and again he speared the balls with an increasing vengeful satisfaction. There, that will show them. There, he could still play golf. There, he was still as sharp as ever. There, still as fast. There, fitter than ever before. No pain halted the movement of his arm, the smoothness of his swing, the rhythm of his breathing as the plastic tube swallowed each ball. He circled to claim the last of them and swung the buggy around. He raised his head up and his eyes were shielded by his peaked cap. He stared straight ahead. As he faced the old clubhouse a cloud hurried away from the sun and caused a beam of light to fall on a butterfly resting on a nettle stalk. The sudden warmth made the butterfly flutter and open the brilliant crimson of its wings that were bordered like a condolence envelope in velvet black. Reg quickly moved his foot from the throttle to the brake. The butterfly took no notice of him but, responding only to the warmth of the sun, fluttered from the nettle to the leaf of a delicately brilliant Flanders poppy bathed in the same warmth. Reg watched in wonder and the lost satisfaction he felt when he hit a perfect shot rose up in him. Joy clutched his heart in a vice-like grip and caused him to gasp an inward breath. He let go his hold on the tube of balls which spilled, rolling away, free on the grass once more. Reg leaned back in the seat. His eyes and mouth opened and were still.

Mr. Tims' Morning

AT 4 A.M., SLEEP LEFT Mr. Tims with a quiet bow as if the dance music had ceased and it was time to move on to a new partner. The two Nembutal sleeping tablets slid out of his bloodstream, through his kidneys and, with an impish glee (Mr. Tims often thought), into his scant urinary output. The urine gave a parting, churlish nip and sting to his skin as it leaked and oozed around his suprapubic catheter that carried its burden into the grimy bag hung down from the frame of his hospital bed. After his first involuntary grimace, Mr. Tims blinked his eyes open to the darkness. His was an optimistic nature. As he slowly shifted his back, guarding in vain against the incoming pain, so also he shifted his mind away from the purpose of the rubber tube that rose from his abdomen to replace the work of his flaccid penis. It had served him well enough for seventy years but now lay shriveled and ashamed, hidden beneath his bloated belly. If he was honest, the burning pain at the tube's insertion was greater than any caused by a shortage of prophylactics as an army medic during his war-torn youth. *Without any of the fun*, he thought ruefully as he shifted once more in the bed and let out a heavy sigh to cover his breaking wind and signal the nurse he was awake now.

Sitting at the desk in the center of the small ward, Nurse Walker heard him. The lamp arched its light down on the desk, but she could make out the silhouettes of the men in their beds curved around her in a wide horseshoe. She bent her head for a last glance at the page and put down her pen beside the picture of the eye she was trying to copy and memorize. Nurse Walker looked out across the desk and gave a little smile into the darkness. She knew Mr. Tims could see her and was smiling back, anticipating her coming to him as a puppy waits for his master, knowing it must stay in order to receive the attentions that are salvation. Mr. Tims had no choice but to stay. He was bound to his bed by the tubes and fluids as firmly as if by a leather collar and lead. Still he waited, his dark eyes twinkling in his face that was made more sweet by the shininess of his completely bald head and skin blown tightly round by prednisone. It had been months since the radiation treatment had finished; his remaining tufts of hair had fallen out, never bothering to regrow. A decision the hair seemed to have made all on its own, but one that did not entirely displease Mr. Tims. Sometimes he would raise an arm and pass his chubby hand over his bald pate, each time touching himself in gentle wonder at his smooth, cool head.

Nurse Walker slipped out from behind the desk, the sound of her crisp apron unfolding as she stood up. Her rubber-soled black shoes were lighter than regulation uniform, and their purchase had been made on a whim. She picked up her torch, pointing it downward so as not to wake anyone else, and went to Mr. Tims, whose bed was centered directly across from her desk in the midst of the semicircle of men who slept as restlessly as nervous camp soldiers gathered for warmth and comfort around the flame of her lamp.

"Hello Mr. Tims."

"Hello Nurse." He gave a boyish smile, half apologetic yet utterly grateful that she had come to him in the night once more.

"Do you need anything?" She asked the question softly, almost vaguely in a manner that allowed him to be slow in his reply. If he chose pain he could receive an opiate. If he chose loneliness she might stay.

"What time is it?" he asked.

"About four."

"How is the studying going?"

"All right. I still get the light and brain pathways all wrong. Sister Alexander spent another half hour going over them with me tonight." For twelve dark hours Sister Alexander circulated through the wards like a calm blue angel watching over the senior student nurses who staffed the wards as well as the patients in their care. From the advantage of eight years more of open-hearted life, love, and education, she well knew the struggle of these last weeks that lead to final exams. Given as much responsibility as staff nurses, this was, in its way, the first and most crucial of their exams. How would each nurse care for her ward and focus on her studies? Sister Alexander loved the senior students and thought that one day, when she and Ewan did marry, she might begin to teach. So far she had resisted the marriage. For her the sharing of purpose and concern for others must be the bedrock of any proposed relationship. Sister Alexander lingered, as angels do, in her mind; however, Nurse Walker drew the conversation back to Mr. Tims.

"Did Mrs. Tims come in this evening?" she asked.

"Oh aye. She was here as usual tonight. She got to hear the carol singers as they came round the ward."

"We heard them too. They were in the hall when we came out of supper and visitors were leaving."

She remembered how she had first heard them—distantly calling into the arched corridor that led from the staff dining room, once the original chapel, to this old red brick tribute to Victorian progress. As she and her friend, Sally, rose from their meal, the high hum became a soprano whisper calling them both until their footsteps quickened and echoed down the stone corridor. The voices of the carolers reeled them in towards the great hall. The choristers' voices faded out of "Away in a Manger," and, taking a collective breath, they turned with one heart to welcome the fresh young night nurses with "Good King Wenceslas." After the first verse, the carolers turned towards the stairs and continued singing to the families and friends who were leaving the hospital for the night. A slim young woman dressed in grey with a muted red scarf as her only Christmas ornament and a young boy still in his school uniform moved towards the visitors and rattled a little red can hesitantly, asking for donations. The pence and pounds collected on these nights of caroling would go to the Friends of the Hospital and help stock the patient trolleys wheeled around the wards by the aged men and woman who, grateful for some remembered kindness, volunteer on Wednesday and Saturday afternoons.

The two nurses, Ros and Sally, stopped for a moment at the mouth of the corridor to the singing of the "Good King." Ros realized that she had always rather enjoyed the teacher king who knew he was both the protector of his page as well as his master. He was a human sort of king, she thought to herself. Ros liked to imagine that if you were a thief of necessity caught in his reign that the Good King might give you a good break. As the Good King summoned his page to *mark my footsteps good and tread thou in them boldly* so the flow of visitors coming down the stairs freely placed coins in the outstretched cans.

The nurses crossed the hall and walked up the stairs, like young salmon swimming against the tide of exiting visitors. They smiled at each other as they heard the clinking of coin into cans.

"Have a good one."

"You too. See you at break?"

"Probably not, I'm going to stay upstairs and study. Mr. Tims usually wakes about that time. I like to be with him now." She did not add that she did not know who would leave the ward first: her to final exams, Mr. Tims to his final rest.

"All right. See you in the morning." Sally turned to the right into Victoria, the woman's surgical ward, while Ros turned left and, climbing two more stairs, swung under another arch, and entered Edward, the male ophthalmic and neurological ward. The older men on this small ward had mostly undergone eye surgery, while the younger were stricken with an array of neurological conditions that were being watched and treated with floundering efforts by young unknowing doctors unable to stop the raging of inflamed neurons that tore through the bodies of these men like horses bolting for home. Occasionally there were patients like Mr. Tims, who ended up here because they didn't fit anywhere else any more.

It was a small, intimate ward, a safe place in which to slip quietly from one world into the next. That had been eight and a half hours ago, well over half way through the twelve-hour shift.

"Mrs. Tims loves the carols. We used to sing as youngsters in the church, under protest, mind, but then we would go out with the Young Farmers group and it stays with you, you know." Mr. Tims sighed and looked up at the window, at the still, black sky aglow only with the faint orange light of the street lamp below. "Aye, it stays with you."

"Are you uncomfortable Mr. Tims? Come forward a moment and let's straighten you up."

She leaned down towards him, and he felt her strong smooth arm reach under his and her other arm circle his back, bending him forward. He smelt her young fresh body and yearned to touch her skin. She was as precious to him as his granddaughter Meg. Instead he relaxed, let her punch and puff up his pillows. He braced his arthritic knees and pushed his feeble, sore heels into the bed. Their joint efforts moved him up the bed and he fell back against the cool pillows and, for an instant, felt the release of comfort.

"Thank you Nurse."

She stood up, paused to relax her back, and looked down on the shiny, round man; she wondered how much more he would endure.

"Would you like a cup of tea?"

"That would be nice, if it's no trouble." They went through this exchange as if for the first time, not as the routine they had settled into over a month ago, but as their first night together. She left his bedside and walked back towards the kitchen. Passing through the ward she looked at the fifteen other patients, with their eyes closed and their minds—where? Mr. Tims so often appearing to be the only one awake, she wondered if there was an unspoken alliance between the other patients to give him this time. Somewhere she had heard that prisoners on death row let the man who was condemned to die with the rising dawn sing alone all night.

The kitchen was warm. At the beginning of her shift, before she even entered the ward, she'd filled the huge tin kettle and put the flame under it on low. Now it glowed a blue welcome to her as she entered the room. Through the kitchen window she saw Venus shining brightly down over the moon, as ethereally round and full as Mr. Tims, she thought.

Nurse Walker carried the strong, sweet cup of tea back to Mr. Tims. His black eyes twinkled as she returned across the ward to his bedside. His pudgy hands reached out shakily in the dark to grasp both the tea and the moment, stolen with delicious sweetness. He sat forward to allow her to plump up his pillows once more and slipped back with a sigh of deep contentment. For a moment all was forgotten as he took a sip of the hot, comforting liquid.

"Listen Nurse, I hear the lorries coming down the hill. It must be a market day today."

"Thursday. You're right." She replied quietly as she too looked out of the window behind his bed to the brow of the Hogs Back Road. One by one the yellow street lights led down into town.

In the next bed, Bill's eyes blinked open. He turned his head towards the pair. Nurse Walker was standing close to Mr. Tims' bed, her thigh resting against the turned cuff of his blanket with a lax intimacy, as if, unconsciously, she also drew comfort from his closeness. Bill stirred restlessly, feeling a jealous pang. Nurse Walker turned her head towards him.

"Good morning Bill."

"Do you think there is a spot in the pot for me?" he asked with a weak grin.

"Of course. Two sugars, right?"

"Thanks love. That'll be lovely."

Nurse Walker looked down at Mr. Tims and their eyes met, smiling goodbye. She left his bedside and walked away through the ward. Now, looking out of the kitchen window across the sink, she could make out the first shadow outline of the cattle market and railway station in the town. Venus lingered in the sky, dimming reluctantly with the rising dawn. She did not switch on the kitchen light.

It Says Love

THE WHIPPET-THIN YOUNG MAN walked close behind the woman into the beauty salon on Parliament Street. To Jennifer's old eyes his physical closeness to her was protective as well as aggressive, and held a threat to anyone who might harm the young woman, for that was his privilege. By the condition of the young woman's eye and the right side of her face it was a privilege he had exercised recently. They seemed to be in their late twenties, and walked both loose and tight together as they made their way towards the middle station of the manicure bench. The young woman sat down while he stood, shoulders bent, over her.

Jennifer sat high up on the big, black massage chair, with her feet in bubbling water, looking and feeling like a pensioned dowager queen on a throne. In her right hand, like a scepter, she held the wired remote control that turned on both the back massage and feet bubbles. It had been over ten years since she had been in a nail salon. This visit was pushed by a gift certificate from her daughter who did not approve of the quantity of gin Jennifer could consume on a warm summer evening and thought that her mother might feel better from a little pampering. At this moment Jennifer's black, baggy skirt was hitched up to her knees. Today she wished for those long ago elasticized knickers into which to tuck her skirt, but any elastic would have been as tight and painful as a tourniquet squeezing her flesh. Her thighs had blown up like late summer marrows and were too visible under the old graying pink knickers that shrouded the dark depths of her sagging pubis. She sat unflinching as little Tula scrubbed the soles of her feet and recited, as if kneeling to a confessional priest, "I have been in Canada for eight years, yes with my family, I am from Vietnam." She said this as a litany every day to inquiring clients. Usually it was enough to satisfy them, but Jennifer was kept young by curiosity and conversation.

Why, that little thing isn't even half my weight, thought Jennifer as she watched Tula take another pumice stone to the bottom of her foot, trying to smooth out the rough edges. Tula seemed to soften into the old woman's gruff kindness even as she scrubbed more vigorously on her feet. To take her mind off the sharp tickling that was close to pain Jennifer looked over again at the couple.

The young woman had got up from her chair and was now washing her hands meticulously at the sink. She turned her hands over and over, moving the soap suds through her fingers slowly, relishing the warmth of the water. Jennifer could see how terribly thin she was. Instead of the usual prick of envy she felt at seeing someone young and slim, Jennifer felt an ache, a long dormant maternal urge stirring for this girl. The girl's posture held no vibrant life force, her body seeming only to stand for survival. For a moment she wondered what it would take to get this young woman to eat a good meal. Maybe a long hot bath would do it; she looks like she could use that too, Jennifer thought to herself. She envisioned the young woman wrapped in an oversized terry dressing gown with her washed hair knotted in a towel sitting in a chair in the sunlight of Jennifer's messy kitchen and herself gently removing the terry turban and combing through that tangled hair. "I'm Going to Wash That Man Right Out of Your Life," Jennifer hummed the tune to herself and was caught for a moment wondering if she had actually been singing out loud. The young woman continued to wash her hands with a repetitive slowness that could appear as if she was preparing carefully in readiness for this needed manicure. To Jennifer it looked more like belligerent sink lingering, and her washing made the man restless. Everyone in the salon was conscious of him staring at the young woman and his movements as he shifted in the seat he had taken beside her chair.

The young woman dried her fingers one by one, as carefully and slowly as she had washed them, and returned, like a dog coming back from a good smelling tree on a retractable leash, to her seat, with small, slow steps. Lulu, another young manicurist from this stable, bent over the young woman's hands for a cuticle check before releasing her to the boss's care.

From a lifetime of watching and being watched, the young woman was aware of Jennifer's observant looks. She had also stared at Jennifer's broad, flat feet that were being grasped first by the toes and then held deftly, like a fresh coconut, by the heels ready for trimming down. The razor blade flashed in its curved handle as Tula swiped accurately at the soles of Jennifer's feet. She skimmed off layers of worn, yellow flesh that fell in a final death dive to the soggy newspaper that lay on the floor between Tula's outspread legs. The young woman wondered if that hurt. She curled her own toes instinctively and wondered again if you needed to be stoned to have it done. Her feet were not where she would choose to apply a razor.

Jennifer's feet were now scrubbed, her toenails clipped and filed, and her legs, to just below the knees, had been vigorously massaged with cream. Tula reached over to the sterilizer and pulled out a pair of pink sponge toe-separators. Jennifer was not happy with the red she had carelessly chosen. It was the rushing of the decision that made it wrong as well as the color. In her dissatisfaction Jennifer absentmindedly picked up a bottle of metallic mauve varnish and looked at it with curiosity. Tula suddenly swung back onto her bottom and raised both her feet up into the air.

"Try mine, it's pretty," Tula said in a confident chirp. Jennifer looked at Tula's tiny but sturdy feet and thought they were surprisingly pleasant. She nodded her consent.

"All right, something like that might be nice." Tula hopped off her stool and brought back three bottles. Jennifer chose one. Tula applied a strong, but not sparkly, red varnish deftly and cleanly to Jennifer's toenails. When Tula finished, Jennifer eased herself off the high altar chair of pedicure heaven and with her feet encased in a pair of blue rubber slippers that had "One Canada" stamped across their velcro top, she waddled across to the manicure bench beside the young woman and her man. Kim, the father and owner of this franchise, was now sitting in front of the couple.

"May I look? Do you mind?" Jennifer asked the young woman as she was getting up. Jennifer kept her eyes firmly on the young woman's face as she asked. How old, how young was she, she wondered to herself. Jennifer dared not look away from the face, though the guarding, hovering presence of the man oozed out a sheet of concern that spread like spilled motorfuel across the floor. One wrong move, thought Jennifer, and this salon would be demolished. The young woman held out her hands for Jennifer to see.

"Do you mind my looking?" inquired Jennifer with uncharacteristic repetitive deference. The young woman shrugged and kept her hands still for Jennifer's inspection. Her nails were long, shaped strongly, and sanded ready for the application of some new kind of beauty. Kim silently held up a sheet of acrylic with transfers on it under the metal lamp for the couple to see. The young man looked very quickly at Jennifer and then away again, his face beginning to show the end of his patience. The young woman spoke lightly, "Not at all, see," and held up her hands.

"What happens now?" Jennifer asked.

"We put these on, we're choosing now." The young woman waved her fingers vaguely towards the acrylic sheet.

"It's all right," she had sensed Jennifer's consideration, "I was watching you too." Jennifer's heartbeat gave a skip of hope for the woman. "Does it hurt your feet?" the young woman asked, looking down at Jennifer's feet and up again at her face.

"No, not at all," Jennifer lied. "And they feel so much better now. What do you think of this color?" Jennifer realized that the woman had been watching her pedicure with some curiosity but was more familiar with other uses for a razor.

"It's pretty," and with a half smile she turned back to the counter and placed her forearms and hands down, spreading her fingers apart for Kim to work on, as she would later spread her legs for another man. With one hand Kim readjusted his angle lamp, pulling the arm closer to him and his goggles down over his eyes. He looked down at her hands, bringing his focus solely onto her nails, precluding the rest of her body. Kim pushed away his imaginings of what acts she would perform with these hands and the nails he was to give her. The young man slid forward in his chair, resting his arm across the counter, closing in on Kim's workspace like a farmer at a country auction leaning across the metal barrier eyeing the animals brought in for sale.

Jennifer waited for Tula to bring the dish of warm soapy water and more polish from which to choose for her manicure.

"That one," said Jennifer. Tula laughed.

"Not the same, too bright? That's OK. This one nice too."

For a while, the salon was quiet. The hum of the traffic through the open door was soothing and distracting enough as Tula and Kim worked side by side on the downhill slope of these clients. Tula was relaxed now. Before Tula had applied the varnish she asked for payment and the old woman had added five dollars, not the usual three that the affluent girls who came in every week usually gave her.

Another group of young people came into the salon, two women and a man. They were younger than the couple already seated and lighter in years and knowledge. One of the women was pregnant. The other woman was tall, thin with black curly hair she had half-contained with a scarf, and she wore bright red lipstick as black-haired, white-faced women can. Her long black summer dress hung close to her body and danced around her feet which were lifted off the floor on thick rubber-soled, thonged sandals.

"Any chance of a manicure?" the tall girl asked the shop in general. Her smile lifted her face to point towards the squared ceiling and fluorescent lights. Kim glanced up at her, his mask hiding the fact that his lips were compressed again at the rudeness of regular customers who did not bother with a phone call for an appointment. It was towards Wendy and another waiting manicurist that he nodded for this group. Soon they were settled and all chatting away and the young man within this group turned his body towards them and held his hands in two bowls of soapy water on the counter while loudly and cheerfully calling out colors for his companions to wear. He loved playing with colors. For him, this Tuesday afternoon on Parliament Street in Toronto was a moment of heaven.

Jennifer's manicure was finished now and she looked at the results of Tula's work with surprised pleasure. For a moment she pushed back her own sense of the waste of Tula's work. Now she only had to sit still and let them dry. How hard, Jennifer thought, it still is, even at this age, to sit still. Tula took away the blue plastic sandals and quickly pulled out the toe-spreaders before giving back to Jennifer her own white flip flops. Any pampering of herself had always felt alien and Jennifer knew she would never get used to it though it was a lifestyle that the young women who came in off the street and out of the suburbs took for granted. She wondered how this family afforded the shop's location and how hundreds of such shops across the cities and suburbs survived. Were manicure salons the new parking lots and dry cleaners for money in need of laundering? She realized that she was an accessory to something she would never know.

The young woman was also finished and getting ready to leave. As she got up from her chair the man rose and stood beside her.

"Let me see, may I?" Jennifer asked again, suddenly wanting one more moment of connection, not wanting this afternoon to end. The young woman flashed her hands with their new, long coated nails pointing downward in front of Jennifer's face as a practice flourish of how she would play them on the bar counters during dark nights like finely knotted fishing flies cast upon fast moving rivers. Diamond and white letters danced through the red blood varnish. Jennifer stared, struggling to find beauty in the brittle talons before her eyes. In one blink her gaze of bewilderment turned to pity that the young woman caught before it was gone. She straightened up her body before Jennifer could speak. The man standing close beside sensed that the old woman had flustered his mare. His lips tightened along with his grip on her elbow as he steered her away from the old woman. He would have to bridle her hard before she settled to obedience again.

"It says 'love'," said the young woman. She looked into Jennifer's eyes with scorn before turning sharply and walking out of the door. The man followed close behind her.

Morning Coffee

"I'M MAKING OATMEAL AND coffee. Would you like some?" Jean looks up at Chris as he stands by the kitchen counter. Her son had arrived by train the night before, taking a quick break from his job in Paris. They had a bare twenty-four hours in which to say hello and goodbye before returning to their separate lives. He answered slowly.

"I think I'll just have coffee. Thank you." Chris goes to the old stuffed chair and sinks into it. His tall frame folds up, making his knees stick out. It is an uncomfortable looking chair but she knew that even with his height it feels safe, enclosing. The oatmeal cooked quickly. The coffee percolated up through the blue ceramic coffee pot Jean had bought from a thrift shop last year. She moves through the preparations in her small kitchen easily. Her son sits quietly, staring forward with bloodshot eyes and looking deeply tired. Never before has she seen him like this, quite so still, not laughing, not getting in and out of her way, helping her in the kitchen.

"How did you sleep?" she asks, as she exchanges the coffee pot for the small saucepan of milk on the hob.

"Not well. I had two big ones. I nearly called out, but thought not."

"I wondered if you would," she replies before she can stop herself. How she had hated that when her mother said those words, never allowing her to have a thought, opinion, or action on her own. She sounds just like her mother and knows it is infuriating.

Jean pours the coffee into two cups, whips the hot milk into a froth for what they called their poor man's cappuccino, and spoons it onto the coffee before bringing the cups and her oatmeal to the table.

"That's lovely, Mum. Thank you." Chris gets up and comes to sit at the table opposite her. But before he can take a sip of coffee he looks away, towards the window. He places one hand on his temple.

"What is it? Another one?" she asks softly.

He stands up abruptly, waving his hand back at her—to be quiet, to let him be—and in three strides reaches the sofa. The light is not so strong in that corner of the room and if he falls or needs to lie down, he can.

Jean sits still at the kitchen table, bearing witness to his usually solitary suffering that occurs with the regularity of a bimonthly menses. He holds his hand, palm outward, to ward her away again before clasping the sides of his head within his fists. She sees his temporal pulse throbbing hard, pushing as if to break the skin and mix a bloody outpouring with the sweat that has already made its escape from his body. He leans forward with his mouth agape. Saliva overflows, as it does in a fearful dental treatment, and glistens onto the coffee table in small viscous pools.

Now Jean quietly goes to him and he does not resist her. She puts one hand high on his back, between his shoulder blades, and feels the sweat that has drenched through his shirt, fresh from this explosion deep within his brain. Slowly he quiets. It is over. Jean hands him a paper table napkin for his face. He takes it and wipes up the saliva from the coffee table instead. He looks up at her, their eyes meet and hold for a brief moment.

He returns with Jean to the kitchen table. He sits down, takes a breath and a sip of his coffee before pulling a pad of paper and a pen towards him. He begins to write a list.

"What are you writing?" Jean asks.

"Names. I'm writing the names of people who live here and I forget. Who is the man who has a new dog?"

"Stan," she says. "Stan has a new dog."

The Museum Visit

BETTY WAS RARELY ALONE now. She had Gladys, whose transition over the years from housekeeper to companion suited them both. But Gladys had taken this holiday weekend off to be with her family. She had prepared and left three meals knowing that Betty would, if she wanted to, enjoy poking around in the refrigerator for more food.

Betty drew her clothes out from the closet and laid them on the bed. She dressed slowly and carefully, checking to make sure there were no wrinkles from her bra, knickers, and pantyhose showing under the smart black wool suit she had chosen. Unscrewing the bottle of Chanel Number 5 toilette, she tipped some into her palm, rubbing her hands together before slowly wiping her throat. She slipped a finger down between her crinkled breasts and dabbed more cologne onto her wrists. The size four skirt slipped on easily and the jacket buttons closed smoothly. She decided against wearing her pearl brooch, choosing instead a pair of angular gold earrings that glowed beneath her bronze upturned hair. She slipped her feet into beige-strapped, low-heeled shoes and plucked from her closet a matching parasol umbrella. She applied her bright red lipstick firmly, outlining a memory where her lips used to be. She resisted the gloves. They dated her. Instead she put on the diamond and gold rings that first Nick, and then Nick's money, had bought her.

She eyed all three black Chanel bags on her bed. They differed only in size. As she often did now she chose the smallest, having need of fewer necessities.

Betty took a final look in the mirror and straightened her back. She pressed her lips together checking her lipstick once more before turning and heading out of the apartment door. The elevator brought her down to the lobby. She stepped out into the brightly lit, marble-floored and wood-paneled space over which hung a huge but simple chandelier. Vernon, the doorman, looked up at her in surprise.

"Good afternoon Miss Betty," he said. "Off out on your own today?" He was not hesitant in asking her such a question although ten years ago he never would have dared. They were both older now. He was stronger and more sure, she less so.

"Hello Vernon. How are you?"

"Can't complain, Can't complain," he replied with a shake of his head, knowing that with Miss Betty there was no sense telling her anything about his life. Some of the others, well . . . some were interested and some downright nosy, but not Miss Betty.

She knew more about him than he realized. She knew he was separated from the mother of his daughter and that he missed them both. Gladys would always fill her in on the basement news if Betty needed some gossip to while away her morning. But today she had other things on her mind.

"A cab please, Vernon."

"Yes Miss Betty. You wait right here and I'll call when it comes." Vernon disappeared through the front doors and stood on the sidewalk while Betty waited in the cool shade of the hallway. In less than three minutes a yellow cab had separated itself from the pack that was moving along at a moderate Sunday pace and pulled up outside the apartment door. Vernon waved to Miss Betty who was already walking towards him. He held the door for her and bent low, helping settle her into her seat while listening for her destination this Sunday afternoon. Vernon knew she was not supposed to go out alone, but he admired the old lady's pluck. She always went out looking as smart as she could. Must have been a looker in her day, he thought.

Betty knew, as every woman of any age who is paying attention does, the effect she had on Vernon and counted on it, as she had counted on the effect she had on men all of her life. Betty leant forward to speak to the Greek cab driver and felt a pulse of excitement, a slow stirring of the same impulse that had put her on a bus to this city over sixty years ago. Again she was alone and ready to adventure out—this time to look back, not forward, into her life. As the cab driver swung away from the curb, out into Fifth Avenue and across to the far left-hand lane, Betty's mind lingered on gentle, distant thoughts of Nick.

Betty had left Troy when she was seventeen. The town streets that held the few stores slid gently into fields guarding tired farms. She had been restless, too pretty and smart for the town. Her presence in a room had the power to confuse the boys at school and bring a flush and stirring to the men she passed on the street. But these conquests held no pleasure for her, only a resigned acceptance, like that of getting an A on a school paper for which she had not studied. She was bored by school, but the power of her body, its strengths and beauty, were to her as curious and awesome as the night sky to a budding astronomer. Finally, with no anger towards Troy or her family, only an address scribbled on a piece of paper by her pastor, she had boarded a train for Manhattan.

She unpacked her bag in a YWCA room and began to look for a job in the city unknowingly gearing up for a war. Betty's complexion and lips held a budding sweetness, as if promising fresh summer fruit. Jack, who owned and ran Jack's Diner on Third Avenue, gave her a job as a waitress. It was not a big diner but the clientele was steady. Customers knew Jack ran a good joint with fair prices and Jack never rushed them if they wanted to linger over another cup of coffee. Betty worked hard. The men enjoyed looking at her though the women glanced at and away from her quickly and left her as much copper as silver on the table. After her first week, when Jack told her she could stay, she asked about the women.

"The women will always tip a pretty girl less but if you play your cards right you can get more." Jack took a cut of the tips. He swept the money up in his hands and stored it for the girls, as he liked to say. Betty learnt to smile at the women. Not the same smile as she used for the men, but one of deference and acknowledgment of their power. Slowly the women began to relax and accept that the pretty girl must need the money too. Sometimes this produced bigger tips, sometimes it didn't.

When Nick came into the diner she did not immediately pay him any particular attention. He was older, as all men are to a seventeen-year-old. He was stocky in build, like the farming men of Troy, with thick, broad hands that could easily pull off a tractor wheel. But the dark hair that covered his wrists dove rather than slipped under his starched white shirt-sleeves, suggesting an arm alive with movement. Nick was in the garment trade, and those big hands were soft, used to the feel of wool, silk, and brocade. He had been married once to a quiet, uncomplaining woman. A pregnancy had swollen his wife to an uncomfortable size and the doctors advised rest. As the pregnancy drew to a close she had gone into labor, suffered a massive stroke, and both she and their unborn daughter died. It had taken three and a half years for Nick to smile again.

As he picked up his life, working to wealth, he avoided remarriage. He chose instead the harsher anonymous bedrooms of a few girls where he explored a variety of sexual encounters to match his mood. Though lonely he never engaged with a woman beyond a night's pleasure and payment.

Not until Betty that is. As she moved through the restaurant, bending her head to write down orders on her pad, walking from the kitchen to the booths, carrying dishes of sandwiches and mugs of coffee, he watched her. Her skin was smooth and radiated the quicksilver vitality of youth. Her hair was soft, a golden color, cut short in an impish bob and held away from her face by a brown pin. Her body was elfin and looked as if it would never blossom into a ripe womanhood. Her long slim legs ended with her large feet that pointed forward as she walked.

For over a month Nick came in and sat at one of Betty's tables.

"What will it be today?" She handed him a menu and set down a glass of water beside his cutlery and napkin.

"Hello, Betty," Nick replied, making a show of pulling his head back and looking directly at her name tag. He had just turned fifty-four, an age where vision slips and words begin to dance in different directions up close or far away. Nick surprised himself when he added, "I'm Nick, you can call me Nick."

"Hello Nick. What will it be today?"

"I'll have a pastrami on rye, and coffee." There was no "What have you got that's good today," from him. Nick responded to her question without looking at the menu. He rarely asked another's opinion of anything. He chose his fabrics by feel and color and his fashion designer clients had come to look at Nick's warehouse of fabrics with interest and acknowledged his eye.

Betty took his order, snapped the menu shut, and walked back to the kitchen counter to call in his request.

What was it that made him look at her a second time? Was it the safety he felt in Jack's cafe? He knew what could happen to young women alone in the city. They could so easily end up "working for a lady and keeping their own room." As Nick watched Betty walk away an emotion in him stirred, not lust exactly, but a desire to care for her and to receive gratitude beyond that of a deal well struck. For a moment he felt as if he were choking. She was looking underfed, and her eyes darted like a small sparrow searching for crumbs in the park. Well, if she was a sparrow, he could play the king pigeon. And with that thought he sat back in his booth and waited for her to return with his coffee.

"Here you go Nick." As she put the coffee down she looked at him and offered another little smile. "You take cream, don't you?" She was trying to remember.

"Uh hum, thanks," replied Nick. Yes, there was not much time, better start right in and see what comes of this. When Betty brought his check he asked her if she would like to join an old man for a drink at the end of her shift. She thought about it briefly. So far she had never been to a bar in the city. Nick was a regular customer and though Jack had warned don't get fresh with the customers, she couldn't see the harm in just a drink after work. She agreed to meet him at Earl's Tavern at seven o'clock.

It had been an easy, steady, and businesslike relationship right from the beginning. Although both of them had been surprised at how much they enjoyed each other's company. Nick was made giddy by an autumn flowering of passion and he powered himself into her with an untapped vigor. For Betty her sexual awakening allowed her to abandon herself to the animal strength of Nick's body. She was in awe of his raw masculinity and his natural ability to draw out her energy. It was not love. Yet it was love. They both knew that their time together would become memories. They would not live happily ever after.

It was six months before Nick had drunk enough of Betty in solitude and realized that if he were to keep her quick mind as interested in him as her young body then he must open up her world. He found her a small apartment on the edge of Greenwich Village and gave her an allowance that enabled her to furnish it in comfort. Having her own apartment, even as Betty understood the implications of her rent payments, made her happy. Nick began taking Betty out with him to meals with his fashion house clients and knew that it would not be long before one would look again at her long legs and boyish figure. He was right. It was two months.

Leonard was a thin man. He had a thin body, thin legs, thin fingers, and a thin nose that was balanced perfectly in the center of his thin face. An hour into their first meeting he asked Betty if she would come to his studio and let him photograph her. She arrived in the afternoon of the next day. Leonard was always pleased when he could find new models himself. Usually Madame Coco chose her own girls which often made them difficult to work with. But the few models Leonard had found were always grateful to him and willing to work—and play, if he so chose.

Betty said goodbye to Jack's cafe and allowed herself to be swept along the fast current of this river. She worked hard for Leonard, while gently resisting his personal advances. He didn't mind. He slept with his girls with a mild sense of curiosity and politeness, to make sure they felt desirable at all times, as much as the pleasure they fed him. He loved the human body, found beauty in every facet of flesh and would, after the war was over, make a living photographing the city's humanity in all its grotesque beauty. Betty had a sense of the rightness of her work both for Leonard and Nick. Leonard had no need to upset the arrangement.

Five years later, after she had returned from a long working week in Washington D.C., Nick's death cry, arching over her that night, had surprised and saddened her. Though Nick's death had left her with a comfortable income, she continued to work. She was not promiscuous until, in the stern of her forties, with her figure intact and the last rush of her estrus flowing, she freely harvested the fruits of her desiring. It had been a grand time. A time of power, a time of pleasure which she embraced with little hesitation.

⚜

At the stop sign the cab driver turned left and made his way back uptown on Madison Avenue. It took a full fifteen minutes until they reached East Eighty-third Street. Although this was a long holiday weekend the big city streets were still crowded with traffic. Only the rich, and the fortunate young who could, had left town. Those who remained were families for whom the effort was too costly and those who cared for the elderly and sick. The elderly themselves knew that for this brief time the city belonged to them as it had when they were young and strong enough to claim it. Another left-hand turn brought the cab to the steps of the Metropolitan Museum of Art.

The driver pulled up to the curb and pressed his meter to stop. He waited for the old lady to open her bag. Why can't they do that earlier, he thought as he suppressed a sigh. He glanced in his mirror to watch her. You never knew with some of these ladies. Sometimes they had no business being out alone and sometimes they just needed someone to talk to and fuss over them for a minute. For that another fifty cents would come his way. Fifty cents for half a minute and a smile was good value, and he knew his worth. Betty leaned forward in her seat. She opened her purse and found the ironed dollar bills inside. She looked again at the meter.

"Five dollars and forty cents ma'am. Can you manage all right?" The driver spoke slowly in case she could not see or hear or even maybe think.

"Five dollars." Betty responded as if she couldn't believe it was more than two.

"Five dollars and forty cents." The driver replied and suppressed another sigh. Slowly Betty counted out six dollar bills and handed them to him through the open window.

"Keep the change. Thank you," she said with the air of a patron handing him a grand prize. The driver released his third sigh. He barely nodded a thank you.

He put her money away, allowing her time to get out of the taxi but not offering to help her. Betty closed her wallet and her purse and felt along the side of the cab door for the latch. Slowly she turned her body and putting her parasol down firmly on the pavement eased herself out of the door. With one hand she clutched the parasol and with the other closed the cab door behind her and, looking straight ahead, crossed the sidewalk to the stone staircase that led to the museum. The ruffles on the parasol fluttered shyly upward. It was only as Betty began the long climb up the steps that the sturdy shaft of the parasol became her cane. She slowly wove her way between the small groups of young people who were sitting about the steps. When she reached the top she gave no outward sign of the breathlessness and racing pulse that shook her frame.

The young dark-skinned security guards who stood behind tables inside the building had long ago given up any semblance of checking bags for serious weapons of mass destruction. Their eyes were downcast and apologetic. They seemed embarrassed as they opened, glanced in, and quickly looked away in one motion sliding each bag back across the table into its rightful owner's hands. With Betty they simply waved her through, leaving her at a loss standing in the large, cool, marble entryway.

Turning to the left, Betty followed the crowd towards the admissions desks and opened up her bag once more to buy her ticket. She drew out two ironed ten dollar bills and was puzzled when in return, along with five sullied singles, she was handed a little green disk. It took a long moment for her to grasp that she was supposed to pin it to herself. Would green go with the gold trim of her black jacket? She fumbled as she attached the disk to her lapel without the aid of a mirror.

Betty lifted her head and held her parasol a little tighter as she moved with the crowd into the grand sculptured hall. She paused to catch her breath and reacquaint herself with its majesty. Light poured in from the huge glass wall and ceiling at the end of the hall. She walked forward slowly, caught up, carried along by the health and strength of the people around her.

To her right, under the massive glass dome rose *The Burghers of Calais*. They stood grouped, paused, locked in their dark anguish, racked weary with the work and responsibility that acquiring money can bring. Forgetting the money that surrounded her in a cocoon of comfort, she stood eyeing these warriors of old with their overflowing bellies. She turned and sat down on a marble bench in front of the cold alabaster statue of Venus. Beauty past and present was before her. She smiled as the crowds of young women passed by. They barely looked up at Venus and never glanced at Betty. She stayed long enough to catch her breath, then, holding her parasol firmly, she rose and walked to where a crowd of people clustered around a small booth and cash registrar. Liz Walton, as her name tag said, stood behind the counter doing a brisk trade in scarves, photographic books, and trinkets to the visitors just emerging from the Coco Chanel exhibit. Betty waited a moment, taking in the size ten suit, until Liz finished her transaction. Liz looked up and leaned towards the older woman who also leaned forward in a conspiratorial fashion.

"Yes, can I help you madam?" she asked. Betty waved a hand in the air and the gold chain swung the little Chanel bag to and fro as she spoke.

"The entrance, where do I enter?" she asked in the brusque, commanding manner of the New York native.

Liz looked over her spectacles at the woman in front of her.

"Down along this corridor," Liz pointed her left arm out. "Turn left through African Art and then left again through Ancient Greek Vases and left again."

"Thank you," replied Betty. "Thank you very much." She said again, pausing, trying to remember all the lefts Liz Walton had told her. She couldn't. She set off down the corridor that Liz had last pointed to and made her way to the African room filled with cases upon cases of warrior masks and spears. She couldn't get a sense from the drift of visitors which way to go next. A young African-American guard was enjoying helping three Japanese students. Betty waited. Only when he had finished with the young women did the guard look towards her and raise his eyebrow.

"Chanel?" Betty spoke the word as a question. The young guard smiled gently in acknowledgment of her solitary journey and pointed behind him and to the left.

"That way madam. The entrance is through there," he added.

"Thank you." Betty nodded her head. Leaving the African masks, she turned left into Greek vases. Hesitant as before a lovers' meeting she paused a moment. She looked at the gold leaf painted on the vases as if taking in the unwanted presence of a guest at a cocktail party while searching for the entrance to her tryst.

The door was sliced out of the wall like a carved rock opening in a cliff face. Betty stared into the darkness and at the sudden crush of people who were standing at the threshold of the exhibit. She took a long breath and entered. A quick look at the introduction written out in careful large black script did not tell her anything she did not already know by heart.

Betty felt a surge of dizziness wash over her. The dark room, the crush of people, made her feel faint, breathless and hot. For a moment she wanted to leave. The fingers of her right hand gripped the handle of her parasol more closely, while with her left she touched and smoothed away the tightening ever present pressure in her chest. The brightly lit cabinets holding the blank-faced mannequins drew her closer. Even in her days of modeling she had rarely seen these early dresses and suits. It had never been fashionable to look back, nothing was vintage then, merely old or new.

But now, as she edged forward to the first of the glass cases, she looked carefully at the earliest creations from this mistress of fashion. Here was the first flowering of Coco Chanel's success, a long black sequined gown that draped with mermaid elegance over the mannequin and was designed to take ten pounds off the most spoiled Manhattan matron. Betty paused in front of the case and pressed her hand down hard on her parasol again, and straightened her spine as she did so. As years ago, from hunger and fatigue during a show, she now willed up adrenaline from her exhausted, withered glands and moved forward, walking slowly down the row of cases. She was conscious of the cool air being pumped into the rooms drawing out the smells of summer flesh. Her nose twitched like an old terrier's on the heath, searching for a faint essence of perfume. There was none. Each case held three to five dresses of a particular period and show. Chanel had so much of her work flowing from one dress to another that they appeared as a continuous bolt of fabric, cross-dyed, cut, and crunched into fluid shapes by the same hand.

Soon came the very successful line of accessories. First it was the glitter of belts and show buckles turning day into night, shining alone on the fabric. Then came the first signature little black bags, so simple in a quilted leather that looked almost soft, but for the gold link-chain handle and clasps. The bags had become instant hits, appealing to the matron who wanted only Chanel in her wardrobe and also to the woman craving just one Chanel dream in her life. Coco had used these bags to reward the models and mark them as Chanel girls when they went out about town. The girls loved the bags, the prestige, and the belonging it presumed.

Betty smiled as she looked at the display of small, medium, and large bags. They were all in one case together at the turn of a row between the 1940s and 1950s. She stood taller with her own bag across her left arm, unconsciously assuming one of the poses she had brought with her to the house as a young woman.

Next, hanging lightly on the size two mannequin were three daytime suits, navy, beige, straight, and pleated. The skirt length revealed the curve of a slim calf and a stylish shoe beneath it. The arms were broken at the elbows, turned at such an angle as to evoke a gesture, a mood, a question, a beckoning, a casual interest but not disdain. Disdain was left for the live models to drop on the matrons of the time.

Betty searched each display case. Her eyes brightened with the recognition of a dress, a name returning, a friend, a rival from her memory. The crowd moved her forward. It was impossible to withstand the pressure of all the people. She had fallen in step behind a tall young woman, wearing torn, taut jeans, big hoop earrings, and with heavily made up black eyes. The girl clung to her leather-dressed boyfriend. Both had long untidy hair, his curled down his neck, clasped in a rubber band, hers gathered in two bunches and perched jauntily above her ears. Neither one noticed the old lady they had caught, following in their wake. They moved slowly forward together until, once again, they paused in front of a case of three evening gowns. The young couple did not hear Betty gasp. In the front was her favorite dress. A full length black evening gown glistening with beads on the folds of the skirt, tiny pleated ruffles from the hips, a widening of the bust line, and then sheer strong lace to cover the bodice and shoulder straps. The mannequin was even poised as Betty had postured. Behind it were two other dresses she remembered were worn by her friends Annie and Jane who had not begrudged Betty the glory of this black gown for that show.

The friends had stayed in touch after they stopped modeling. Both Annie and Jane had married well and remained on the East Coast. After Nick died they had included Betty in social events when they needed an extra pretty woman. Jane had died a few years ago in Boston, but Annie still lived with her husband in Philadelphia. Betty stood looking at the gowns, remembering their friendship. Suddenly she was tired. She clutched her parasol with both hands and felt she had to move or she would fall down. She looked around for the young woman and her boyfriend but they were now far ahead. Betty wanted to call them back to her, to show them these dresses, to tell them of the friends she used to have. But she knew that, at best, they would only nod, fix their eyes on her face and listen politely. They would not hear her story as any way their own.

She breathed in, holding tightly onto her parasol as someone jostled her from behind and moved her forward into the brightly lit gift shop that ends all exhibits. She looked over to Liz Walton who was still busy at the cash register with women pushing and shoving to pay for books, mugs, and key rings that would never have crossed the desk of Chanel. Betty held her bag closer to her side and made her way through the crowd into the main hall and the exit. She stepped outside and breathed in the hot muggy air of her city.

The steps down from the museum to the street were still crowded with contented young people, many drinking water or soda from plastic bottles. Her young couple—Betty had come to think of them as hers—had gone, diffusing out into the park woodland as captured fish swim away when released back into the lake.

Betty peered downward in order to place her parasol on the step. She felt shaky and vulnerable as she moved slowly to the bottom. Only on reaching the pavement was she able to straighten her back once more and look for the bus stop. The number five would take her home. She wanted to linger still in the company of strangers and stood close to a middle-aged couple who were also waiting on the sidewalk.

It was three minutes before the bus came and swayed to a stop outside of the museum. The couple who had been standing in front of her stepped back so she could get on ahead of them. She was weary, shaken, and yet not quite ready to quit. The bus driver was patient with her fumblings, as she tried to deposit the correct coins in the machine, before she sank into the seat designated for the elderly, close to the driver. The bus moved away from the curb with a swish and a rumble that spoke of its city efficiency. After the first stop Betty had regained enough breath to look about her and take in the avenue and park as the bus passed by. She looked forward anxiously to each cross street waiting for her own. The bus stopped almost outside of her apartment building.

Vernon was still on duty in the lobby. He lifted his eyebrows when he saw Betty step off the bus and cross the road by the traffic lights. She looks tired, he thought, and, yet, there is a fresh flush about her too. He held the door open in readiness for her as she climbed the three steps up to him.

"Welcome back Miss Betty. Did you have a good time?"

"Yes, thank you Vernon." Staring straight ahead she walked passed him to the elevator doorway. Leaning hard on her parasol she pressed the button and waited for the elevator to arrive and take her back upstairs.

Spring Fever

FOR OVER TWO WEEKS now female gray-haired relatives—daughters, daughters-in-law, granddaughters, and nieces—had been stepping off the elevators carrying bunches of bright yellow daffodils. There, Gwendolyn knew she was right. It was spring again. She could always tell. She loved the scent of new beginnings that she caught in small snatches as the flowers dripped their gooey sap onto table tops before being captured in vases where they withered and died in two, maybe three, days. The fresh air that also accompanied the nurses into the building hung on their uniforms like dew drop fairies and she could breathe in the fragrance as it lingered through the first of their shift's rounds. Their uniforms did not feel cold as in winter, or smell fetid as in summer but were fresh as in new, and hopeful, and willing.

Gwendolyn had been ninety when she broke her hip. She remembered the fall. Her son Jonathan had been visiting, unburdening himself as a schoolboy drops his backpack on the kitchen table coming home from school, about some unsettling business that he always brought her. If he had found a wife he could have shared his problems with her. But he had never quite had enough courage to overcome his fear of rejection by even the mildest and sweetest of women, and he had never dared approach any other kind to make that leap into intimate companionship. Most mothers would be glad, she supposed. She had never been that maternal and, though she had loved him the most of her children, was a little disappointed in him. He could have got on with his life and made something more of himself than owning a furniture store. Admittedly it was his own store, not a franchise, but though she had tried she had never become excited by his work or his world and found it, and him, rather dull.

Now she was in a place of her compliance but not choosing. After the fall and surgery she had suffered her first heart attack. On leaving the

hospital she had been brought up to the twenty-first floor from her apartment on the third floor of the Willow Ridge Retirement Home for Seniors,
though there can't have been too much wrong she thought with satisfaction. Between the crossword puzzle solving minds of her doctors and the
seemingly endless variety of medications they prescribed, her heart kept
its own discreet rhythm. Some days all she felt was tired—other days not
quite so. Her mind kept on working but the energy needed to gather and
share her thoughts often seemed more than she could spare. Her hip had
not set well. She was now bed and wheelchair bound and that is what kept
her up on the twenty-first floor, the dying floor. You weren't supposed to
call it that but everyone knew. When you came up here from downstairs
your absence was missed by your friends who met for lunch in the dining
hall. They inquired after you for a week at the most. Maybe even a few
brave, staunch friends came up to see you but nobody could stomach it
for long. The beds that were made with hospital linens not your own and
the half-filled urine bags that hung down from them spoke of another
intrusion into the body. The visibility, through doorways always held open,
of a friend's barely covered nakedness, was all too stark a reminder of the
possible future. Everybody knew that this could be their last home. If they
were lucky they would die in the bed they moved into but the chances of
that were not high. Nor, truth be told, were the odds much better for dying
in the building. You had to be quick about this dying business. Gwendolyn
had seen it time and time again. Someone came up here sick, got a little
better, sometimes even got to go back to their apartment for a while, but
others were not so lucky and lacked the strength or desire to return to life's
circus. If the nurses caught them at it, slipping out of bed to the floor or an
unknown realm of consciousness, then off they were sent to the hospital
across town and with luck, for the staff, died, having had everything done
to keep them alive, over there.

After three months the nurses got used to the fact that Gwendolyn
would not get well enough to go back to her apartment, and accepted her
as one of the long timers. In the mornings they bathed and changed her,
got her up into her wheelchair, chatted about breakfast that had been and
lunch that was to follow. But they rarely spoke of anything that occurred
outside of the ward, either past or present.

Gwendolyn's son Jonathan had been relieved when his mother decided to sell her small home in Baltimore and move to the Willow Ridge Apartments Retirement Home for Seniors in Philadelphia. Willow Ridge was about an hour's drive from where he lived alone in the city and he had been able to visit his mother there regularly, twice a week, for the last fifteen years.

But when Gwendolyn had taken her fall and had her 'turn' as she called it, he had not expected her to recover. As he was unmarried and the geographically closest of her children he assumed the main responsibility for her care. He phoned his two sisters regularly and they took turns coming to visit at least once a month. One lived in Southern California, the other in Arizona. Both sisters had raised young families and though they now had more time to pay attention to their mother, they were happy to leave the primary responsibility to their brother who, they both thought, deserved it. As children they knew he had been her favorite, so now he could at least do this for all of them. Gwendolyn was seen by physical and occupational therapists twice a week but they merely filled up the hours of the day rather than engaged her or improved the health of her body or her mind.

Gwendolyn's husband had died of overwork and sadness in his early sixties. She had cared for him tenderly as loyal wives do and she had not remarried. Too old by those day's standards and realizing that time was now finite she did not wish to care for those men who came calling, shopping, with pensions and money plans to bargain, sniffing her out as a good caretaker for their last years. She was not lonely. She had been lonely enough in her marriage and now relished a solitude that was free of any matrimonial or maternal guilt. After her husband's death she allowed herself the extravagance of adding annual flowers to her small, sensible, suburban garden and to pursue a mediocre golf game, enjoying the female companionship it afforded her. Now, at ninety-two, she was thankful for the strength that those pursuits had given her mind and her wrists.

But Gwendolyn's bones and muscles were too fragile to bear her weight and when she had been given a wheelchair she quickly learned how to use it. She had made that adjustment more easily than either she, her children, or the staff could have expected and was soon able to move around the nursing unit with surprising agility for someone of her age. She needed help getting in and out of the chair but that all came under the nurses' care plan for her well-being.

"Gwendolyn bathed, dressed and up in her wheelchair," was in her daily notes. She was such a fixture, in fact, that she had become an easy patient, or client as patients were now called under the more advanced economically efficient care manuals. She was often assigned to young student nurses when they rotated through the unit as part of their expanded practical experience. Under the gentle guidance of Viola, the nursing aide who had cared for Gwendolyn as long at they had both been on the twenty-first floor, these young nurses approached Gwendolyn cautiously. Her stick-thin frame and apple ancient face made them tentative. Most of them had not yet a familiarity with the physicality of aging. They reached out to touch her gently as if she were an antique porcelain vase that they might break if they were clumsy. But she would look up at them, her gummy lips quivering around her now oversized loose false teeth, and smile, letting them wash and hold her. Often they would ask, in the condescending, nervous voice of the young who instinctively know that they have no right to such presumption, "Would you like to wear your pink or your yellow blouse today?" Gwendolyn would point at one or the other, but truth was, she didn't give a toss just as long as they would get her up, and dressed and in her chair.

It was the springtime arrival of daffodils which seemed to transfuse their oxygen into her blood so that desire rose in her like the sap of an old tree, urging her to go downstairs and sit in her chair on the steps of Willow Ridge looking out across the man-made city lake and just one more time greet this season of birth. She continued this vigil in the hallway during the long hot summer months even when the air-conditioning sucked out the sweet smell of putrid body waste. But as summer faded into autumn and the days shrank to a low winter light, her body would feel the changes. Her bones ached more and told her that it was no use. For the winter months she would remain fairly quiet and compliant as the nurses wrote with relief in their notes, "Gwendolyn up in her chair today. She sat quietly in the corridor."

When the weather was storming outside she did not even wheel herself down the corridor to the elevator. The smell of wet raincoats depressed her and reminded her somehow of her married life, working and walking home from the bus stop laden with grocery bags that disintegrated in the rain.

But in springtime she returned in her wheelchair to the open hallway between the elevator and the nurses' station to breathe in the freshness from the nurses and visitors as they came in from downstairs. Slowly the smells of the outside world built up in Gwendolyn's memory. Her mind collected in its own vase all the spring fragrances of the bouquets brought in until by Easter-time she could stand it no more. On these days she would wheel herself down the corridor to the elevator doors and sit there.

"Good morning Gwendolyn, up early today?" The oncoming nurses might smile at her but sigh inwardly, knowing that with Gwendolyn up and in position so early this might be a difficult day.

When the elevator doors opened and a new visitor stepped out Gwendolyn edged closer. The unsuspecting visitor would smile, admiring the determined little old lady's independence, and perhaps hold the doors open for her. One of the nurses would look up from the station, strategically placed close by the elevators, and with a patient, thin smile, grab the back of the wheelchair.

"Where do you think you're off to Gwendolyn?" they'd say, and then pull the chair back into the hallway to let the embarrassed visitor make an escape down the corridor to their loved one who had ended up on this floor. It can't be that bad, they might think to themselves as they hurried away. Gwendolyn never answered the nurse's query. Everything but her room, number two thousand and thirty-three, and the corridor were denied her. She sat silently in her chair, a hand maybe now raised to her chin or both hands folded in her lap, submissive as they placed her further away from the elevator. She would spend an hour or so sitting in the chair each morning and then take herself back down the hallway to her room to wait for lunch at noon. The amount on her tray for each meal was more than she had ever eaten or served to anyone in all her years as a wife and mother. She picked through the food carefully, having long ago given up any guilt about the waste that might feed the starving in China or Africa or wherever people were starving today.

One morning, Viola came into her room smelling of the jasmine that she brushed against on her daily walk to work. Viola was small and dark-skinned with gray straightened hair, a sweet smile and a limp that somehow signaled a wordless understanding of the Gwendolyns of this world and her place beside them. She recognized the determination in the whiskered chin that Gwendolyn thrust forward and upward to ward off the world even as she was being dressed to enter it. Gwendolyn was happy to see Viola pull out her mauve sparkly sweater with the three-quarter length sleeves. When Gwendolyn was all ready for the day, Viola pushed the chair into the corridor, past the utility rooms, onward towards the nurses' station. She was up early this morning and no one was at the desk. All the nurses were with patients or hovering around the one or two doctors who came with a hurried efficiency to the floor. Gwendolyn positioned herself in the empty corridor and waited, watching the visitors and staff coming and going. She stayed there through the morning, returning to her room for lunch.

During lunch, rain began to fall. She could see it out of her window. It was a soft spring rain. When she woke up from her nap, she looked across her bed out of the window, and saw that the rain had stopped. There were clouds in the sky yet the sun was shining sharply as if examining the blue canvas on which to paint a rainbow. The afternoon still seemed fresh and to hold a lingering promise. Viola came back into the room and changed the diaper that Gwendolyn wore all the time now before setting her in the wheelchair once more. Slowly Gwendolyn wheeled herself down the corridor again and positioned herself in front of the elevator to watch the new shift of staff coming on duty. Each nurse, as she got off the elevator, eyed Gwendolyn warily. The change of shift was a busy time while both crews of nurses were preoccupied with the shift report.

Today was especially busy. After seventeen years at Willow Ridge, Viola was retiring. The nursing supervisor had come down to make a speech. A handful of purple balloons were tied to nursing charts and bobbed up and down uncertainly. A large square chocolate cake covered in butterscotch cream had been brought in inscribed in blue icing with "Goodbye and good luck Viola. Thank you for everything. We will miss you."

The party noise held Gwendolyn's attention. She remembered parties of her own life. Celebrations of birthdays, daughters going to college, friends at work, marriages, and even her husband's funeral. She sat alone by the elevator, lost in memory.

Because of Viola's goodbye party the allotted half-hour for report ran on and both shifts were getting restless. The supervisor had given her small speech but now she was ready to go. The day shift was anxious to leave and the afternoon shift was ready to begin their work. Patsy, the head nurse, made a tentative gesture at clearing up the mess from the party but, as she always had, she left the main body of work for Viola to do herself. Viola took the leftover cake and carefully slipped it into a smaller box someone had found. She would take it home for her sons, who, though grown, still stopped by to graze out of her house. Viola hardly thought about this final leaving. She had been thinking about it for over a year, counting down the weeks and days and she was ready. The pain in her arthritic hip had been constantly with her now for five years. She limped from the nurses' station to the locker room and began putting her things into her bag: an extra pair of comfortable shoes, a hair brush, never-used toilet articles that a patient had given her as a Christmas gift. She threw some old magazines into the waste bin in the locker room. The box with the remains of the cake was tied up with the balloon ribbons. She walked out of the locker room and passed the nurses' station.

"Goodbye Viola. Come back and see us soon. Don't forget us now," Patsy called out as she too began to gather her belongings. Viola smiled to herself.

"I surely will," and knew that she would never return. She walked across the hall to the elevator doors. As she pushed the down button she saw that both elevators were busily delivering and unloading staff to and from other floors. She turned back to see Gwendolyn sitting in the wheelchair, watching her.

"Goodbye Gwendolyn. You take care now." Viola smiled at the old lady in the wheelchair, who paid no attention to her but looked straight ahead at the elevator. Viola moved behind the chair to smooth and absentmindedly straighten the old lady's hair. On an impulse Viola bent down to give Gwendolyn a kiss. Just then the elevator doors opened and two groups of visitors got out. They were laughing and happy and young. Gwendolyn stared straight into the now empty space. Viola also looked up into the opened elevator whose fluorescent lights blinked from inside, beckoning like a fairground ride, at them both. A long-buried instinctive remembrance of escape made Viola grasp the handles of the wheelchair and push it into the elevator. Quickly and expertly she turned it around to face the door, put on the brake, and pressed 'Lobby'.

The doors closed. The elevator slid smoothly downwards, by this time of the day smelling faintly of pureed meals and baby powder. There was a stop at the seventh floor where another tired attendant got on. She exchanged nods with Viola but said nothing. The elevator reached the bottom floor and with a gentle swish the doors opened.

Three hundred and fifty pound Marvin looked up from his desk, saw the wheelchair holding Gwendolyn, and sighed. He already had his hand on the phone to call upstairs before he saw Viola pushing the chair out into the lobby. She had placed the box of leftover cake on Gwendolyn's lap and the five purple balloons bounced and bumped together in the whirling breeze from the revolving doors.

"Good afternoon ladies. How are we doing today? Can I help you there?" Marvin raised his huge body up out of his chair and with the surprising grace of the morbidly obese, slipped past the wheelchair to the door and held it open. Viola deftly steered the chair down the ramp of the arched entryway.

"Thank you, Marvin."

"Is Jonathan not coming today then?" The question hung lightly on Marvin's lips.

"We'll be back later," responded Viola and she turned the wheelchair to the left along the pavement towards the lake that lay glistening before them. The air was fresh and a little cold. Viola reached down to pull Gwendolyn's sweater more closely around her frail body.

Gwendolyn looked straight ahead as they crossed the main road and reached the beds of daffodils bobbing their yellow heads. The tulips blooms were just beginning to blush crimson from the moss green of their leaves. The breeze shook pink cherry blossoms and sprinkled them on the pathway. The ducks swam their broods towards and then away from the new arrivals to the lakeside path. The breeze rose and danced into a wind that whipped the pathway dry from the rain. It blew the clouds away from the sun-spattered rainbow that shone across the far end of the lake. Gwendolyn breathed the chilled air deeply into her old lungs and smiled.

Phone Calls

LISA LOVED THE EARLY morning stillness which greeted her when she took fresh water and feed to her hens. She loved opening the henhouse door, standing back to watch the leaders fly from their night-time perch and dive into the run for the grain and treats she scattered. This first morning chore always eased her into the next, of dew-laden harvest. Now, in April, the last of the Tuscan kale lay alongside the early fava beans and a full brimming box of pink-red rhubarb. Lisa chopped the rhubarb leaves short like a child's summer Mohawk hair cut before carrying the boxes of bundled, shining vegetables to the back porch-bench. She sat down beside them, one hand silently stroking the wet kale before leaning over and taking off her grass-spotted boots, then padded into the quiet kitchen to brew her first pot of coffee for the day.

Bob was with Sam, who had picked him up as the sun crested over the last dawn-grey cloud. The brothers had driven the twenty-four miles up the coast to the little cove where they kept their old Boston Whaler fishing boat. Sam swung the truck into the gravel parking lot and the two men got out to join the group of half a dozen other fishermen around The Crusty Coffee Shack that served as their start and meeting point.

"Mornin'."

"Mornin'." Greetings were exchanged as they walked towards the coffee shack run by Sandy, the only woman at the cove. She watched the brothers come towards her and noticed again, that while the twins had still carried their twinness into late middle age, Bob was definitely losing weight and color. His face was no longer tanned and ruddy, but grey and yellow under the rough stubble that the men all wore on fishing days.

"Mornin' boys. How ya doing? Coffee?" Sandy's call was cheerful and strong.

"Mornin' Sandy. Yup. Two dark and strong will do it." Sandy turned half away from the men and as she poured their coffee into large styrofoam cups, asked, "How's Lisa then?"

"She's doing all right. Off to The Sea Surf Lodge and Rock Isle View today. She's got more than a couple of crates to deliver. Not bad for this time of year."

"Good for her. If we did real food, we'd be buying too."

"Well, you do real coffee Sandy. How about filling her up again?"

"Right. Here you go." Sandy reached out across the counter for Bob's styrofoam cup, pulled it towards her and refilled it to the brim. He nodded his thank you. Her eyes held his, inquiringly for a brief second, the unspoken questions: how was Bob feeling today and, as importantly for Sandy, how was her friend Lisa? She found no answer in Bob's face.

The brothers turned away from the coffee stand and walked over to join the other fishermen on the tilting dock at the water's edge. The sea was ruffled—wavelets toying, still undecided whether to rise up in a temper or fall back into calm. The men sipped their coffee and looked out. They followed the forecast but always they learnt more when they stared out at the sea.

Sam turned to Bob, "That should do it." Taking final sips from their cups they flipped them into the garbage can while walking to the truck and gathering up their gear: rods, reels, buckets, chum, an extra gas can, and coolers. Sam reached into the cab, collected his radio, checked his cell phone, and locked the cab of the truck.

"Have a good one boys," Sandy called out to the brothers as they walked back along the dock. She began to tidy away the mess from her early morning coffee customers. Since opening The Crusty Coffee Shack five years ago she had become an unofficial harbor master. The cell phones have changed things a lot and she doesn't feel so connected to the fishermen she had come to call her boys, still it was with her that families left messages, looking for husbands and brothers who were out longer than felt safe and whose cell phones were out of range.

Bob climbed into *The Sea Urchin* and reached up to take and store the tackle that Sam handed to him. The routine between them was easy. Even though they got out barely once a week they were good fishermen. *The Sea Urchin* was primed ready to go, the refill gas cans pushed into place on board, the coolers of bait and beer stowed in their places, the rods and tackle stacked and racked ready for work. But Bob was sore and breathless by the time they were done. Gathering himself Bob turned the ignition key and the engine throbbed and growled into life, sounding strong. Bob looked over his shoulder at the water churning out from the two engines slung low from the rear of the Boston Whaler. It wasn't a large boat, medium in size and horsepower. The brothers had bought *The Sea Urchin* together ten years ago, after they had crossed that threshold into middle age and their bodies had begun to crumble from the contracting work they had pounded at and had pounded back at them, for thirty strong years.

The Sea Urchin bobbed and chaffed in the water. Sam had let her loose and was gathering the buoys and ropes neatly away.

"All set," Sam called out.

"Here we go," replied Bob, and slipping the gears into reverse, he gently guided *The Sea Urchin* away from the dock, turning her until they faced the open water of the bay. The boat moved out into the dancing water, cresting each wavelet eagerly as if she were a barely contained young thoroughbred filly easing into the starting box at Bay Meadows race track. Bob's hand on the tiller held her steady.

The two men stood side by side, looking ahead. They loved the roll of the bay and the fraternal roles the *Urchin* assigned them. It was as if they were boys again, following the path their father had led them. Bob was the older of the twins by three minutes. He had always led, bossed, and watched out for Sam. The rhythm of their lives had brought success and happiness in equal measure as disappointment and sadness. Five years ago the loss of their father had been followed, a year later, by that of their mother, teaming their parents in death as they had been in life. And this last year it seemed that Bob had slipped sideways and fallen in a trajectory of his own. Bob's discomfort had become more than indigestion, it became abdominal pain and after many doctor visits and tests Bob was wondering if he had a clinging Sea Urchin of his own.

The *Urchin* motored steadily across the water, whose choppy beginnings had calmed to an easy rocking as they knew it would.

"The Point I think," Sam said.

"Let's give it a try." Bob upped the revs and the little boat motored on for another half mile before they turned to face the sheltered inlet beside The Point. Sam dropped anchor and let the boat rock in the water. The brothers set out the rods and threw chum over the weighted lines. It was barely midmorning when Sam reached into the cooler and brought out the first couple of beers. Cracking one open he silently handed it to Bob before reaching for his own and they took their first sips of the day. Sam looked over at his brother, waiting for the lines of pain on Bob's face to soften, just a little.

Lisa finished her coffee and tidied up the kitchen. There is not so much to do now with just Bob and her at home. Their two daughters drop in and away again like young fledglings, returning, squawking, to their familiar hole in the roof. Since Bob has been having his tests they come by more often, taking turns watching their parents. They don't yet know what it means but can sense a shift in both Bob and Lisa—a gentleness towards each other that had not been present since before the girls' adolescence that had nearly torn the family apart. Both girls had been difficult, pushing the boundaries of the small home and family with their yearnings. Lisa thinks of her daughters as she runs water over her mug, holding it tightly between fingers and sponge. It is early enough in the day that she could light a forbidden cigarette and there would be no trace of it lingering in the home when Bob returned.

After wringing out three wet dishtowels Lisa takes them outside and drapes them over the boxes of beans, kale and rhubarb. She opens the hatch of the Subaru station-wagon and places the boxes carefully in the back, leaving the rear windows and the hatch open while she gathers up the rest of her things. She climbs in and starts up the car.

Lisa has a self-imposed limit of a twenty-five mile radius for deliveries of her produce. The Sea Surf Lodge is only ten miles away. By the time Lisa pulls off the main street and parks the car close to the side entrance Manuel has propped open the screen door for her. Somehow he always seems to know when she is coming and is always there, gently ready to help her.

"Buen día Manuel."

"Buen día Señora. Como estas?"

"Bien, muy bien, y vos?" Each time she sees him she practices these few phrases with perfect pronunciation but gets no further with her vocabulary. They smile at one another. Lisa carries her boxes inside and lays them on the counter. Stacy, the dessert chef, comes out, happy to see her.

"Hi, how have you been?"

"Terrific, thanks. Oh that looks fantastic. We never saw rhubarb like this at the Union Square market. I'll get the beans to Brin. He'll like those."

"Great. Hope you have fun with this. Here's the bill."

"Thanks, I'll take it back to the office. OK with a check later?"

"That's fine."

Just as Lisa turns to leave, Stacy asks, "How are you doing? How's Bob?" The question is beginning to come more often as concern spreads like mushroom spore through their gently woven community. Lisa pauses before she answers. She really doesn't know how her husband is. The tenderness that is growing deeper between them has not yet stretched to truth telling beyond the few facts that they know: Bob has pain, the pain doesn't leave, there is blood, and the doctors order more tests as the months continue.

"He's feeling pretty good today. He and Sam have gone fishing."

"Oh that's great." Stacy smiles in relief at some good news. "Make sure he keeps Ted and me in mind if that boat fills to overflowing." They laugh together.

"Will do. I'll check in next week?"

"Please. This is great but I bet I've gone through this box by Wednesday."

When Lisa leaves the restaurant Manuel is nowhere to be seen. Lisa makes one more delivery at the Rock Isle View before turning the Subaru homeward.

It is almost lunchtime and she is hungry. She didn't have any breakfast and so can justify the two thick slices of bread she toasts before smothering them with peanut butter and strawberry jam. Sitting down at the kitchen table she pulls the day's mail towards her, sifts through and registers how quickly the doctor bills keep coming. She puts those to one side and reaches for the *Hobby Farms* journal. She is trying to focus on an article about baby carrot and has just finished the first slice of toast when the phone rings, jarring her from her break. She goes to answer it, leaning against the stove before she speaks.

"Hello?"

"Hello. This is Doctor Marks' office. Is Mr. Baker there?"

"No. This is Lisa Baker, his wife."

"Could you have Mr. Baker phone us right away. Doctor Marks wants to see him as soon as possible. His test results are in." The voice manages to say Doctor Marks in a way that distances the voice from being anything other than the messenger. Lisa can't summon enough strength to respond and is silent for a moment longer before saying, "He's out fishing with his brother. I'm not sure when they will be back."

"Can you try and reach him? It is important that he contact us today."

"I'll do what I can. Thank you."

"Thank you." The voice on the other end is softer and Lisa is grateful.

She presses the phone down hard on the receiver, stopping herself from trembling. She feels nothing. If later someone were to ask her to define "feeling numb" she would look back at this moment as her experience of numbness. She makes her way back to the table and, sitting down, repeated the conversation in her head, going over each short sentence that the voice had said. They want to see him. Today. That is not the phone call of "everything is fine." That is the phone call of "something is going on." She got up and, reaching for the other mobile handset phone, sat down. She dialed Bob's number but only hears his receiving message. She tried Sam's but the same thing happens and she knew they were out of range, maybe as far as The Point. She dialed Sandy's number at The Crusty Coffee Shack. Please, please, silently she urged, please, please pick up.

"Hello," Sandy's voice came briskly down the phone line.

"Hi Sandy, is that you?" Lisa's relief coats her words.

"Lisa? Hi, yes, Sandy here. What's up? How are you doing?" Sandy slowed her questions, knowing instinctively that Lisa had not phoned just to chat.

"Are the boys back yet?" Lisa guessed the answer but didn't know how else to start this conversation.

"No, no one's in yet. I heard on the radio that some boats are having luck out there. They have all gathered past The Point. I guess Bob and Sam started out there."

"Oh, no wonder they can't hear me, out of range, again." And Lisa gives a nervous little laugh. "I'm wondering, can you reach them? Bob's doctor's office phoned," Lisa takes a breath before saying out loud words she doesn't want to hear. "They seem to want Bob to call in right away, and go to the office if he can." She dare not say any more.

"Sure. I'll try. Get them to head to the office from here when they come in. Shall I call you at home when I reach them?"

"Yes please do. I'll be at home."

"OK. I'll call you as soon as I have any news."

"Thanks Sandy. Bye." Sandy looks at the phone in her hand. That's not good, she thinks, and hanging it up turns to the radio to reel in those boys.

⁂

Lisa sits back, listening to the silence of the empty afternoon. It could be a while before Sandy reaches the boys with the radio or they come into range with their cell phones. She stays away from busying herself on the phone. She wants to be by the phone but not on it. What could she do? None of the chores that wait with endless patience calls out to her. The laundry, the dishes, even the recent mail all lie dormant. She needs to be able to get up, do the dishes, and prepare the evening meal. She sits still before idly turning the radio on to the local station for the classical afternoon hosted today by her friend Susanna. The afternoon opera music and Susanna's voice soothe her. Lisa looks out of the window and watches the pair of starling parents fly back and forth to the barn feeding their very hungry brood whose three open mouths stick out of the siding. Years ago Bob had sliced into the side of the barn with the pick-up truck and chipped off a small chunk of wood siding. He had always said he meant to fix it but had never gotten around to it. Lisa suspects that for all of his grumbling he enjoys the starlings as much as she does. A sunbeam moves through the window warming first her legs and then her body, softening the outer edge of her tension. She closes her eyes until the phone rings sharply, cutting through the soft music of the radio.

"Hi Lisa. It's Sandy. I reached the boys." She laughed. "They didn't want to come in. They are all having a great day out there. Everyone is on a run and looks like they will get their quota. I did what I could but they may be having too much fun." Lisa laughed her relief. That they were fine, always a worry, and even that they were baulking on coming in.

"Ask Bob to call me after he has been to the doctor's office. It's quicker for him to go straight there than come home first."

"OK. Will do. I'll call you too."

"Thanks. Bye." Now Lisa could move. It would be two hours at least before she heard anything more. Stuffing the handset in a pocket she got up and went outside. In the shed she picked up a shovel. She needed to dig deeply, rather than rake softly.

⚜

It was Sam who pulled *The Sea Urchin* up and called time.

"That's enough for us today. Lisa won't be wanting more in that freezer of yours." Bob nodded. After Sandy had reached them on the radio he was ready to head in. The tide was with them and *The Sea Urchin* made good speed back to the dock. The brothers moved with the same methodical purpose as always; cleaning up the boat, washing her down and leaving her shipshape ready to take them out again the next time. They carried the rods and tackle and two coolers, one now empty of beer, the other heavy with cleaned fish, onto the dock and made their way back to the Dodge truck. Sandy came out of the back of her shack.

"Good morning boys?" she asked, though she already knew the morning had been good.

"Heading north?" Another question, more important than the first, Sam looked at Bob who looked away, out to the sea.

"Yes. Might as well." Bob let the words fall from his mouth as if a beer can was slipping through his fingers. And added as if to himself, "It's time to go."

"I'll let Lisa know you are on your way then." Sandy wanted to keep them on course.

"Thanks." It was Sam who answered. For now that Bob had said yes he too wanted to be on the road.

"Bye now. See you boys next week," Sandy said, though this time she was not sure if she would.

Sam and Bob stowed their gear away in the back of the pick-up and climbed into the cab. Sam eased the truck into reverse and swung out of the parking lot and up to the road. Sandy watched and breathed a sigh of relief when they turned north and headed up the road into town.

Back in the house Lisa's phone rang again. She knew to pick up the handset and sit down to answer.

"Hello. Hello is that you dear?" She was quiet as she listened to Bob.

"I'm on Sam's phone—mine's gone dead." He laughed nervously before beginning to tell her what the doctor had said. The words spilled out of him. All the unspoken thoughts and fears they held, singularly yet in communion, were released as he spoke and she listened, letting him pour his heart into hers as he had his body. She received him still. Let him spend himself in all the telling and all the fear and all the knowing and unknowing. Finally he was silent.

"We're heading home now hun. We'll stop at the market. Is there anything you want?" Lisa's heart lurched—yes, oh yes, there is much that I want. She replied, "Yes. Yes, I think so. I want ice cream. Bring back some ice cream—and chocolate."

The Waiting Room

NO ROOM WHERE SOMEONE might enter was ever left in darkness at The Hospital of the Holy Angels. In the surgical waiting room on the third floor the low lights under the cabinets shone down on the counter and desk, waiting for Joanna to enter at 7.45 a.m. Joanna switched on the overhead fluorescent lighting, making the room stir, rouse and show itself ready for her inspection and the start of a new day.

She put her purse in the cupboard behind her desk and stuffed her knitting bag into one of the lower desk drawers. She had signed up for a double shift and this was going to be a long day. She checked the chairs and little tables while laying out two copies of the local daily paper, the A.A.R.P. monthly magazine and *Your Hospital Stay*, an in-house brochure about the amenities to be found in the Holy Angels. It was the reading of last resort. Her clipboard lay beside the telephone. Next she unfolded, smoothed and spread out another copy of the daily newspaper on her desk. At 7.55 a.m. she was prepared for her shift, half an hour after surgery began every weekday morning at The Hospital of the Holy Angels. The morning's routine was familiar for the medical, nursing, and auxiliary staff, but never so for the anxious patients or their fearful relatives.

Joanna was sitting behind her desk when the door to the waiting room first opened and Carol arrived, alone.

"Hello. Am I in the right place? Mrs. Oaks, waiting for Mr. Oaks." Carol's bright smile did not cover her confusion. Joanna, looked at her clipboard though she already knew that Mr. Oaks was first on her list. Her tone gave some comfort as she replied, "Yes. You can wait here. The cafeteria's on the first floor."

"Thanks." Carol looked around at the brightly lit room, seeing nowhere to hide. She chose her seat with care and put her coat on a chair beside her.

The door swung open again and Mary entered. She did not stop at Joanna's desk but walked straight over to where her friend Carol was sitting. Joanna did not mind.

Carol's laugh in greeting her friend Mary was sharp, loud, and nervous. Carol had watched her husband Jack's apprehension grow with each passing month that he had struggled with increasing pain while the arthritis, like a voracious parasite, had burrowed into and eroded his hip joint. Though Carol came from one of the tiny islands off of Vancouver, and Jack the big city of Calgary, it was Jack who carried a deep distrust of, and Carol a shaky faith in, physicians.

The surgical waiting room at Holy Angels had been subdivided, like land and time, out of a bigger room. The old surgical waiting room had held two large sofas, a grouping of single chairs and coffee tables where families who waited there for long hours, coming and going with cups of coffee, bad sandwiches and not enough to occupy their hands and minds, could feel that an effort at comfort had been made on their behalf. There used to be a small chapel to one side, furnished in a sparsely Christian manner, for quiet contemplation by the most devout or desperate of families. Now the chapel had been moved to the Intensive Care Floor. But this waiting room, refurnished for today's economy, had only twelve upright chairs, separated with three small tables, lining the walls. The chairs were one grade up from those in the emergency waiting rooms: they were wooden, not metal, with scotch guarded fabric seats. Easily uncomfortable after an hour and a half, they produced a physiological disease making everyone anxious and ready to move on. The small tables had room only for a cup of coffee and a purse or a sandwich but not all three. Carol had already glanced through *Your Hospital Stay* and learned what care she and Jack should expect in the next few days. She didn't believe a word of it. By the time Mary arrived Carol had given up trying to read. She had put the newspaper back down on her lap and started picking at her fingernails.

"Good job we won the hockey, or the whole game would have been a waste of time. And you know how Canadians feel about wasted time." Carol laughed again, glad to have something light to pretend to care about.

"That's right. I forgot, last night was the finals." Mary was neither Canadian nor a sports fan. This winter's Olympics had passed her by as the rain storms had swept down on her small farm and threatened to wash out her first acres' planting of young apple trees.

"Yes, it was exciting. We watched the game last night, a good distraction before bed, and this morning."

"How is Jack doing? Any news?" Before Carol could answer Joanna glanced up from her paper and responded, "They are just getting him ready to go in. They should be starting any minute now." Both Carol and Mary looked up, startled and staring before they remembered to smile. The name tag, pinned on the upper left-hand side of her pink nylon jacket, read Joanna Kruger. Underneath her name were the words "Surgical Waiting Room Volunteer."

"Thank you," replied Mary, in her most professional voice. She looked at Joanna and wondered what she had been in her life before she was a hospital volunteer. Whatever it was, Joanna was the one in control now. Joanna knew her place, safe, behind her desk. She was the guardian of information. Now she shared her powers of observation, "You are Canadian," she said to Carol, "and you," she turned to Mary, "are English." She spoke the words in a flat voice, as if repeating normal vital signs during a nursing shift report.

"Yes, that's right," laughed Mary. "And you?" she held the question, already guessing the answer.

"I am German," replied Joanna, thereby equaling all three of them as older first generation European immigrants, no different in their yearnings than those of the young people who now scrambled and crawled into the country nightly from the south. There was a momentary pause before they politely connected and compared dates of arrival into the United States. Joanna had come first in 1956, Mary in 1958, and Carol in 1962.

Their conversation paused while a new family of three entered the waiting room. The husband was in a wheelchair, already a white identification bracelet was strapped around his wrist. His wife hovered beside him, her full, plump body soft and unsteady. She held tightly onto a metallic cane as she walked. They looked too old to be the parents of the daughter who listlessly followed them into the room.

Joanna rose from her chair, leaning over from behind her desk and placed one hand on the arm of the wheelchair, corralling the husband by her side, while she waved his wife and daughter to chairs up against the wall. They obediently sat down. The wife looked across the small but significant space on the carpet between herself and her husband now parked beside Joanna. She turned her head around, and smiled at Carol, "Here we are," said the smile. "Here we are again, waiting our turn." Then she spoke, "We've been here before." Carol smiled back a weak hello.

A young nurse, already dressed in blue scrubs, topped and tailed with her paper hat and shoes, came into the waiting room. She carried a clipboard of papers and after checking in with Joanna bent over the man in the wheelchair.

"Hello Mr. Swartz. Can I see your name bracelet?" Mr. Swartz obediently held up his wrist to her. The nurse read his name and checked it against her papers and then said, "Your birth date?"

"August twenty, nineteen thirty-seven."

"Right knee, isn't it?" Mr. Swartz nodded but did not speak. He was beaten. He knew he had failed his body, dismissing its cries for constraint in every way since youth and before age had begun on its path into and through him.

"Are you ready? Off we go." The nurse turned and began to push his wheelchair out of the room. Mr. Swartz raised his hand, the bracelet moved slightly on his wrist as he waved to his wife. Mrs. Swartz grasped the handle of her cane and tried to get out of the chair but couldn't. Her daughter, sitting beside her, twirled the dial on her iPod. She was engrossed in the music that thinly escaped from her ill-fitting ear-buds. Mrs. Swartz waved back at her husband from across the patch of carpet but neither one spoke. With one hand the nurse pushed open the door behind Joanna and with her other hand maneuvered the wheelchair-bound Mr. Swartz through the opening. The doorway swung closed behind them. Mrs. Swartz turned to look at Mary and Carol who had been watching the departure of Mr. Swartz with rapt attention. Carol turned back to this other wife, "Off he goes then."

"Yes. It's his knee. We've done the hip." Mrs. Swartz gave a small laugh.

"My husband is just having his hip done." Carol said it firmly, denying her husband's body any further deterioration while in her care. Joanna looked down at her clipboard that had been updated by the nurse who had taken Mr. Swartz away.

"Mr. Oaks is in now. They have begun work on him."

"Thank you," replied Carol. She was not too sure what she was saying thank you for. Suddenly she wanted to know why they had only just begun on her husband when he had been gone at least an hour. Was she thankful for the information that "they" were working on him now, was it a relief or did it bring up imaginings of her husband, blanched pale by the operating room lights while half a dozen gray-blue-gowned figures surrounded him? Each one pushing and pulling his leg apart from his torso, as expertly as she would twist a chicken's drumstick away from the thigh before dinner. She shuddered.

"Come on. Time for a coffee. I missed breakfast this morning." Mary stood up. Clutching her cell phone in one hand and her purse in the other, Carol followed her friend. They each picked up their coats from their chairs and made their way out to the elevator.

"Oh yes, you have plenty of time." Joanna spoke from her seat behind her desk. No conversation was private in this room. She overheard every one and entered as many as she could.

The two friends walked into the hall, smiling at each other with their mutual amusement at Joanna. Mary pushed the elevator button. They did not have long to wait and rode back down to the first floor and continued to follow the painted blue line leading to the cafeteria. In the cafeteria the server, Carla, was shifting a few breakfast hard-boiled eggs around and adding salads for lunch even though it was still early morning. She knew the staff she served and it was for them she prepared the counters and set their dishes out in rows. The visitors would come and go, spending one or, at the most, three days grazing silently, not sharing any gossip or daily news. Only those for whom the vigil became long and dangerous learned to smile hello as they passed along the line and then to say a thank you to Carla at the check-out till.

The women bought two coffees and Mary plucked a yogurt and a fruit bowl for them to mix and share. They sat down at a table overlooking a shaded courtyard not yet warmed by the day's sunlight.

"How are Bonnie and Mike?" said Mary.

"Fine. Bonnie is coming over later when Jack gets out of surgery."

"Good. That's good. You will be together then. And Mike?"

"Mike called early this morning to speak to his dad. It was good to hear his voice." Mary nodded and sipped her coffee. Neither woman had much appetite. They finished half of their coffee and left the unripe melon chunks in their bowls. Rising to leave, they threw out the bowls, cups and spoons before heading back up to the third floor and the surgical waiting room.

Their seats were still vacant and they reclaimed them with the possessiveness of college students after the first day of class. Mrs. Swartz and her daughter were sitting in their same chairs. Mary took her coat off and laid it on her seat. She walked over to the door with a bathroom sign on it that was behind Joanna.

"Is this all right to use?" she asked.

"Yes. Of course." Joanna nodded but did not look up from her desk as she spoke. Mary turned the door handle and entered another, smaller waiting room, probably sliced out of the same space as the room she had just left. She turned her head slightly; the room didn't need a wide sweep to take it all in.

There were two big shelves filled with sealed surgical supplies. The shelves were beside another door that she guessed led directly into the surgical suite. Two chairs sat with their backs to one wall. These were covered in blue plastic that was easy to wash off after a gowned patient had soiled them. All this Mary absorbed quickly as she went to the bathroom. The bathroom was a patient's bathroom with side rails on either side of the toilet and a call-light cord hanging within easy reach of anyone in the small cubicle. It was when she came out that she saw the simple crucifix, and noticed a third chair, brought up to face the other two whose backs were to the wall.

She blinked as the scene opened up before her. Relatives would be ushered quietly into this room together. Asked to sit down while the doctor stood, before asking permission to sit, in case he might want to touch them. He would sit in front of them, his back guarding the surgery from where he had come, leaving the mess of failure behind.

"I'm so sorry," he would say. Mary imagined a he. "We did everything we could. There was nothing more we could do." And the relatives would look at him, not at first understanding, then not allowing his voice into their minds, before the words pushed themselves forward, rushed in and consumed the brain, darting into every crevasse, covering every convolution, until there was no other thought allowed but that "What he is saying has changed my life forever."

Mary blinked away the scene, opened the door and returned to the main surgical waiting room.

Carol was now calmly reading the local paper. She had settled into the waiting. Her overt worrying had receded and the news of the local high school football team was enough to occupy her mind for the moment.

"Code Blue 345. Code Blue 345." The voice over the intercom held just the barest hint of urgency. Its owner was well trained: "Don't shout, don't panic the visitors." Mary looked up. Code Blue was always serious and they were on the third floor.

Joanna looked up too. Her eyes flickered, but she quickly recovered her composure before announcing to the room at large: "Heart attack. That's a heart attack." Joanna looked around to see that everyone had heard and understood her words. All hearts in the waiting room skipped a beat. Her own heart too, the thrill of commanding such attention, even for a brief moment, was a lift to her day. Carol and Mrs. Swartz looked suitably nervous. Mrs. Swartz's daughter remained unmoved while she twirled through another playlist on her iPod. Assuming an air of calm Mary reached into the bag beside her and brought out her knitting. It was a small portable project, a sock, one she kept handy for these moments of waiting. Now she pulled a strand of wool from her bag, arranged her needles and began to knit. Carol glanced over at her friend and then returned to the newspaper. Home economics was an area where they parted as friends. Mary loved to fuss over the little things, experimenting with decorating cup cakes and had joined a knitting group. Carol would never knit a scarf or bake a cake, but with a spade in her hand she could turn over her vegetable garden in a morning.

Joanna looked up from her newspaper. She passed over the sports section which never held her attention. She liked to spend time poring over the obituaries, searching for names of friends, acquaintances, and even a name that had been on her clipboard in the previous few weeks. She watched for a few minutes as Mary's fingers worked the wool and needles.

"You knit the English way," she said. Mary looked up and smiled.

"Yes, it is how I learned and I could never make the change to continental. Do you knit?"

"Yes."

"When did you learn?"

"When I was a child."

"Me too. I learned when I was young. But I didn't knit for a long time after. Only when my mother became ill and she taught me again." Joanna nodded her understanding of a woman of a certain age whose life duties expanded to the caring of her parents.

"Do you knit now?" Mary continued.

"Yes, some. I knit."

"Where did you learn?"

"I learned at home during the war. We knit as children. Our mother taught us."

"And my mother too." Mary stopped short. A memory suddenly strong in her mind, of the air-raid shelter deep underground, the noise and the counting out loud of the stitches with her mother. The counting, like breathing, stopping them from screaming. The two women looked at each other with an understanding of the age they lived in. They were joined by their flight from old Europe to the adolescent America and a new life. Each woman silently tightened her lips against memory. Joanna glanced back at the paper, Mary returned to her knitting.

The door behind Joanna opened and the nurse who had taken Mr. Swartz away came back into the surgical waiting room and walked directly over to Mrs. Swartz. She stood in front of her and said, "Mrs. Swartz, would you come with me, this way, please." The nurse reached out a hand to Mrs. Swartz who had suddenly begun to tremble. Carol looked up from the newspaper which now fluttered in her own shaking hands. Mrs. Swartz fumbled for her cane. It clattered to the floor. The nurse reached down to pick it up and gently hand it to her. The daughter looked up slowly, suddenly aware that there was a change in the routine of her father's surgeries.

Mrs. Swartz was standing now, shakily holding onto her cane. The nurse took hold of her other arm to steady her as she led her to the doorway behind Joanna. The daughter pulled off the ear-buds of her iPod and followed them.

Mary looked up to see a doctor enter the room from the far door. He stood waiting for Mrs. Swartz to come in and sit down. He opened his hands and began to speak. Mary heard him say, "Mrs. Swartz," before the door was closed to the waiting room once more.

The Vigil

PROTECTED BY INTENSE RESIDENT doctors and experienced nurses during his internship, Peter Gough had managed to avoid it. He had never been the one who looked up and called, "That's it." But his few early memories of sudden death still left him chilled with fear as if at night he was standing on the edge of a mesa cliff facing an unknown drop into oblivion.

Peter had been a tentative boy and grew to become a cautious young man. He had lacked the courage to disappoint his parents and withdraw from medical school. But Peter did love to talk with people and was a good listener. He was a tall, impressive-looking man. Walking through the wards in his white lab coat he carried an air of authority and safety for many patients. For others it was his ordinary kindliness that reassured them. In the 1960s when patients were beginning to look again for doctors who could care for and treat their cold, diabetes, twisted ankle, and angina, he quickly found his place in a small general practice in Northern California.

Peter met Linda at a graduation party where, drunk on relief and cheap beer, he had slipped onto and into her body as a starfish clings onto a rock in a turbulent sea. Over the next six months she became the anchor to which he returned when he was swept away in the currents of stoned craziness through the sixties. He never really recovered, carrying a deeper melancholy with each decade and from the eighties to his retirement Peter changed practices frequently. For all his calm exterior and gentle demeanor he was not a steady man. His patients and coworkers no longer found in him the security they longed for. It had been Linda who raised their three wild children. She painted when she could, capturing a few harsh landscapes as her own. She even sold a few pictures and the small amount of money that came her way was always welcome. She was an outgoing woman who made friends and connections as easily as Peter lost them. During his difficult times she was always able to find one more practice that needed his help for a few months. In this way the years passed. They fell into retirement with no safety net of financial security which a physician's wife could expect as her due after the long years of struggle, worry and loneliness. Linda bore this as well as she had the preceding forty-five years of marriage.

※⊙◎◐※

He wakes suddenly, startled, unsure what has woken him. Not his, nor her, snoring, no it is something else. The bed is shaking. Lying flat on his back he pulls the sheet up to his chin with both hands. His body shivers. His scrotum tightens and shrinks. He blinks and makes an effort to return to consciousness. The bed continues to move and Peter realizes that it is Linda herself who is bucking in seizure and causing the bed to shudder. Peter's eyes lock open and he sits up. Leaning on his right elbow he reaches out with his left hand, switches on the bedside light, and pulls himself into a sitting position. He finally turns to face his wife.

Linda is lying on her back. Her head thrown back, her eyes wide open with the pupils rolled and fixed. Her mouth is clenched shut though spittle is bubbling free from the left side of her lips. She continues to shake.

Slowly Peter's fear fades to understanding that Linda is having a serious episode, but what is it? In all his years of doctoring he has never witnessed these primary events. He knows only the aftermath, the loss of motion, speech, or life. Alone and in his panic he reaches out for the phone and lifting the receiver he presses the large lit numbers, nine—one —one.

The young man's voice on the other end answers promptly, asking first for Peter's phone number and zip code. As Peter replies, 626-1412 and zip, what is his zip code? 98774, the dispatcher types this information into the computer and asks Peter more questions. His tone is efficient. He is tired and only just holding his weary impatience in check. The pager goes off at Clays' bedside. "Medical assistance needed, 182 Poplar Way." Clays lives in the next street over from Peter, and is at the house in less than five minutes. When Peter sees the lights of the truck rise over the hill and pull up his driveway, he leaves Linda's side and goes to open the front door.

"Hello Peter. Where's Linda?" Clays asks as he walks past Peter and into the hallway. Already in his mind he can imagine what has happened; a stroke, and the old boy doesn't realize it yet, he thought.

"In the bedroom. This way," replies Peter. But Clays is already striding through the house following a childhood memory of after school visits with Peter and Linda's children. They all grew up together in Thornton. Peter and Linda's kids had left, pushed out by their mother in any direction but that of their father. And they had all made it out, Pete Jr. into business, Gail into real estate, and Scott to the Sierra mountains. They were making a good living though Scott, the one to take the mountain road, lived more gently. But Clays' parents had not pushed him away. At first they worried that he didn't want to leave but slowly they understood and accepted that his heart beat strongest in Thornton where he found his place in the community he loved.

Clays found plenty in the town to keep him interested. He was curious about the sea and land that surrounded Thornton. He had an old-fashioned respect for the elders who had chosen to stay and live out their lives here. Perhaps, if his upbringing had been in the suburbs, he would have felt that bland constraint and studied to become an anthropologist, but he had no need of that in this community. Here life was lived openly for him to see. He was barely out of high school when he began to train as a volunteer in the local fire department. His path opened up before him and became him, as any wilderness trail did when he hiked in the national park that surrounded their village like a cloak. Here was a way to work with his strength, his community. The following year he enrolled at the fire academy where he met other young men like himself who did not yet realize they were joining a brotherhood that stretched across the continent. Training was hard but he had no real difficulty passing his exams to graduation. Not like some of the others who came with their brute strength and a penal sense of guilt or hope to lift them out of lives that had harsh endings. It was here that he learnt to teach and in teaching relearnt his own lessons. On graduation from fire acadamy he continued on into paramedic training. Only then did he emerge, ready to be posted to communities that he could have grown up in, and they were as far away as he would travel until his retirement twenty-five years later. It did not take long for him to return to his town of Thornton. John, the chief, was ready to hang up his fireman's jacket and it was a natural choice for the town to vote in and hire a young one of their own. They had raised and nurtured Clays and he would care for them when their time came. It was understood.

⚜

Now Clays is striding quickly towards the bedroom and Linda. He cannot remember a time when she had not been in his life. She had been a friend to his mother when Liz had come to the town, a young, bright, brittle hippie redhead. His mother had found her way to Linda and Peter's house, bringing her son to play with their rough older tribe. Linda had baked oatmeal and chocolate chip cookies, made the best lasagna, allowed them to play Atari, Dungeons and Dragons all weekend long, and even driven them to the movies, staying through the show before bringing them home again. Now Clays is here, fulfilling his unspoken debt and promise to her, which would include watching over Peter when this incident was over.

By the time Clays reaches the bedside, Linda is deeply unconscious. Bubbles of foam still overflow from her mouth with each exhalation. Her cheeks are flushed but her lips are the purple blue of a beautiful umbilical cord, the color of birth as well as death. The flashing lights of another fire truck bob up the driveway. Peter goes back to the front door to let Matt in, although he too needs no direction. In Thornton everyone knows their way around everyone else's house with a mixture of memory and instinct. There are few surprises.

Clays has already unpacked his bag when Matt joins him and the two men begin to quickly assess Linda's condition, airway, breathing, circulation, calling numbers, writing notes. Another truck arrives, Michael and Joe show up half asleep. They are not needed and hang lightly, assuming the posture and place of the back-up team, standing at the foot of the bed with Peter who has thrown an old robe over himself. He is not dressed but covered. Clays turns to him, "We are going to have to transport Linda to the hospital Peter." Why does that language always overtake him he thought. "You probably realize what has happened here." Clays defers to the old doctor as he does to all doctors.

Peter blinks. "A stroke?" he says.

"Probably," responds Clays. But in fact Peter has no thought at all what it might have been that caused his wife to buck and shake, rupturing the core of their bedrock, and left her lying on the bed further away from him than she had ever been in childbirth.

Clays radios ahead before driving the ambulance with more care than speed through the country roads to the local hospital. Matt rides in back monitoring Linda and steadying Peter. The night is quiet and an hour later Linda is in the emergency unit of Sunview Hospital. Peter sits beside her, watching the nurses and listening to the beeping of the monitors. He looks at her face, unable to read the machines with enough knowledge to give him comfort.

It is David Block's first week of emergency rotation. He pushes back the flimsy curtain and enters the cubicle. He looks first at the monitors, then at Linda and finally at Peter.

"Hello. How's it going?" He doesn't wait for an answer from Peter but stands, looking at Linda's clipboard and the beginnings of a chart in his hand. A nurse comes in, smiling tightly at Peter and then speaking quickly to Block, calming him, Peter realizes, just as he too had been calmed by nurses. It was the nurse's assurance, his quick movements, a male nurse, Peter blinks at that realization, that makes his gut tense as he watches the men work in tandem around his wife. For the moment they have shut him out, are focused on her in a way he hardly remembers being. Finally the nurse turns to Peter.

"Maybe you would like to wait outside for a moment. The firemen are still around. They want to know if you need anything." Peter stands up, and Block glances up at him, grateful that the husband is leaving. Maybe he can finally figure out what to do next. He too is a tentative physician and will eventually find his way into dermatology. But for now he must focus on the situation in front of him. The nurse parts the curtain to let Peter out and then turns back to help the young doctor stabilize this patient and send her on her way.

Peter stumbles out into the hallway. Clays and Matt come up to the old man who, thinks Clays, looks as if he is about to stroke out himself.

"How's it going in there Pete?" He put his hand on the old man's shoulder and waits for a reply.

"Not too sure," replies Peter. "The doctor is with her now."

"Would you like us to stay? Mike and Joe have the other rig back in town and as long as they don't get called we can stick around for a while."

"No, I'll be all right. Well, would that be all right?" The words come out in a confusion of thoughts as Peter realizes he doesn't know what to do. Clays leads Peter to a couple of empty chairs in the waiting room and they sit down together.

"Where are the family, Pete?"

"The family?" Peter struggles to understand who Clays is talking about. Then he realizes Clays is asking about their children. "Oh, well, let me see." He searches his memory, trying to recall where his grown children are at the moment. Slowly it comes back: Pete Jr. is in Texas, Gail in New Mexico, and Scott somewhere in the Sierra mountains. As he tells Clays their whereabouts he realizes that Clays is looking to see who would be able to come home. Come home. Why did they need to come home? Is Linda's condition that serious? For the first time he realizes it could be.

Less than half an hour later David Block reappears, looking for Peter. The nurse, Bill Love, stays with Linda, busy arranging her transfer up to the intensive care unit on the fourth floor. David is relieved to see the firemen with Peter. It is less frightening to tell relatives bad news if they are with someone. If they are alone there was no knowing how much they will need from you, if they will fall on you, even the men. He has seen it happen. Peter stands up, as if on trial in the dock. Clays stands too, unsure how the old man will take the news he is pretty sure is coming from the young doctor.

"Doctor Gough, I'm afraid your wife is very ill. As you probably suspected she has suffered a large stroke. We are going to admit her to the intensive care unit. The next twenty-four hours will be crucial for her, if she is to (he just stopped himself from saying eventually) recover." He went on. "We will take your wife upstairs now. Maybe you could go to the admissions department and fill out the paperwork. Then you can come up and see her again." He pauses for a moment and is about to leave when he remembers to ask, "Have you any questions?"

Peter isn't sure. He isn't sure what he heard. He knows what the words are of course, but what do they mean?

"No. No questions. Where do I go?" He looks up first at the doctor and then, when he sees that the doctor is already leaving, to Clays.

"Here, I think I remember the way." Clays again put his hand on the old man's shoulder and together they walk out of the emergency room, down the hall to the admitting department while Matt returns to tidy up the ambulance. The paperwork doesn't take long to complete but Peter is grateful to have Clays beside him. When it is all done, the young lady working nights at the desk gathers her files together, picks up the phone and dials the intensive care unit. She speaks briefly before hanging up the phone. Then, with a bright smile at them both, she says:

"There, you are all set. You can go on upstairs. Your wife is in intensive care, unit 421. You can see her now."

The men thank her and stand up. They find their way to the elevator and take it to the fourth floor. Outside of the intensive care unit Clays stops.

"Pete, this is where I have to leave you. Can't go on in there with my beeper and I'm still on call." Peter stands rigidly beside Clays, outside of the intensive care double doors. Suddenly he is paralyzed with his old fear, terrified to walk forward. Clays continues, "I've got to get back now. You will be all right, won't you? You have my number? I'll call Carol for you if you like. She can reach the boys, let them know what is happening and find out when they can be here. One of us will come over in the morning and see how you are doing. You'll be all right, right?"

Peter manages to nod and mutter, "Thank you. You've been very kind. Thank you. Yes of course, I'll be fine." As Clays turns to go Peter takes a step forward. The automatic doors swing open and he has no choice but to walk through them. Clays watches from the elevator and shakes his head. Poor old fellow, he thinks, I hope he will be all right for the night. He glances down at his beeper and sees another red light flashing.

Peter continues to walk, hesitantly, through the doors to the intensive care unit which, even before dawn has begun, is filled with light. A nurse glances up at him and says, "Doctor Gough?"

"Yes," replies Peter.

"Your wife is in bed C, over here. We've put her in this cubicle for now. You will have more privacy. We are close by if you need anything." She gives a brief smile as she walks Peter to Linda's cubicle. She is in a hurry. Linda is the second admission of the night and has remained unresponsive. But, still, the unit is quiet enough that she is willing to let Peter stay.

They reach the cubicle and enter. Linda is lying on her back. An intravenous tube feeds into her arm, an oxygen mask covers her nose and mouth, a blood oxygen saturation gauge is clipped to her finger. As Peter glances along the length of her bed he sees a plastic urine bag fastened to the side rail and realizes Linda has become a silent vessel for the monitored fluid passing in and out of her body. The nurse quietly draws up a chair and motions Peter to sit down beside the bed.

"I know you want to be with your wife. Let me know if you need to go to the waiting room. You can rest there too. Will your family be joining you soon?" She speaks kindly to Peter. He nods at her, unable to reply.

"I'll leave you then. I'll be in and out. My name's Mary by the way. Just ring if you need anything." She turns and leaves the cubicle so smoothly that Peter does not notice her go. He turns back to Linda lying in the bed. Linda is breathing deeply and slowly. Her face is flushed through pale shades of pink yet despite the oxygen mask her lips remain blushed blue and purple. Her features are relaxed. There is no sign of tension or struggle about her face. As he sits down he feels no panic, only a deep, tired peace. He draws the chair closer to the bed. Gently taking her hand in his he bows his head on them both and begins to vigil with her through the night.

Doctor Patel
Comes to Tea

"GOOD MORNING JANE." DOCTOR Patel strode past his secretary's desk not looking at her as he entered his office and closed the door behind him. The moments of transition, driving from the psychiatric hospital where he made rounds each morning, enabled him to shed the images, smells, and sounds that pricked at his senses and lingered in his clothes after leaving the wards. He loved the unknown, uncharted pathways that his patients seemed to be traveling back into their brain. Like an archaeologist surveying the workers on a dig he would sometimes linger on his walk through his wards, searching for the occasional shard of memory to be shaken free from the rotten decay of dementia.

He turned back to his desk and sat down with a sigh. He reached for his pile of correspondence for the day, and began to read Doctor Frank's letter. Doctor Frank had written a brief outline and history of his care of Mrs. Andrews and asked would Doctor Patel be able to see her and sort out some kind of diagnosis and suggest some management. The letter closed with the normal thank you and then Frank had added, *I think you will find her interesting.*

Patel put the letter down and thought about Frank. The two men had met when they were in their psychiatric rotation at the Clearwood Hospital. Their paths crossed often again as they set up practices in the same county. A friendship between the two men had begun to germinate in the hothouse enclosure of the locked male ward at Clearwood but the exhaustion of the workload had thwarted their efforts and the budding companionship had no time to flourish. Besides, both men were somewhat shy and quiet. Frank was conscious that his comprehensive scholarship and brains had got him into medical school, while Patel was one of an ever-growing Asian medical presence that was still outside the core of young men and women who considered entrance to medical school their right.

Patel swiveled his chair around to look back out of the window at the gray, cracked parking lot with the unshaded cars baking in the sunshine of this English summer morning. He saw his old Honda Accord and winced as he felt its paint blistering in the heat. It was a useful car for home visits, more functional than prestigious. He gazed over the flat roof of the old barracks that had fallen into civilian use. After fifty years nothing had been done to lift the austerity of a necessary post-war mentality. Even the buildings' names still conveyed their royal, nationalist origins: Alexandra, Victoria, Elizabeth. Funny, they are all women, all queens he mused, though he had never bothered to explore why that was. He reached for his phone and dialed Mrs. Andrew's daughter, Maureen King.

"Hello?" her voice a question.

"Hello, is that Mrs. King? This is Doctor Patel."

"Oh yes, oh, hello." He heard her surprise at his unfamiliar voice.

"I am phoning about your mother, Mrs. Andrews. Yes, I would like to come and see her today, this afternoon, after my clinic is finished. It would be about five o'clock. Would that suit you? I am sorry it would be so late." He spoke quickly as he always did when he had already decided what would work for him.

"Actually it would work out quite well." Not very well, don't sound eager and say very well, Maureen thought to herself.

"It might be between five and six tonight. You are sure that is not too late?"

"No. That will be fine. Look out for the beech hedge, that is the entrance." But it won't be fine, Maureen thought.

Sadly she realized that Doctor Patel was right to visit her mother in the evening and see her at her worst. A night's rest allowed oxygen to flow to her mother's brain and bring brief moments of clarity and articulation in the morning. But as the day wore on and she struggled to stay mobile, to stay in control, the synapses of thought and speech closed like flowers at the end of the day and could connect no more, leaving her brain to strike out on its own down the pathways of old memories and new paranoias.

Maureen knew that the woman Doctor Patel met that evening would not be the same one who would come to greet her when she arrived to visit in a half hour's time.

Maureen and her mother began their visit, as they always did, with a catch-up cup of coffee. Maureen cupped her mug in both hands and said casually, "A Doctor Patel is going to come and see you this afternoon."

Mrs. Andrews moved a little forward in her chair, no longer relaxed, watchful, wary, and a little bit excited.

"Who is this doctor?"

"Do you remember Doctor Frank wanted another doctor to come and see you? This is the one. He phoned to say he would like to come today, after he has finished his clinic, so I don't expect it will be before five, probably closer to six, but he still might like a cup of tea." Maureen stressed the time of his visit and knew that she would have to repeat it again during the day if her mother was not to feel surprised by his arrival that evening.

Her mother sat back in her chair taking it all in. She sensed another challenge—another predator coming to stalk her in her nest. Why couldn't they leave her alone, she thought, both women thought. Why must she be hounded and hunted, flushed out into the open to be sniped at as she stood vulnerable, old, and losing her mind.

Maureen said nothing more about the new doctor's visit for the moment.

Instead she asked, "What shall we do about lunch? Would you like to go out?" Maureen was relieved that she could provide some distraction to the challenges that lay ahead.

The fish pie at The Princess was always hot, cheesy, and comforting. They both sipped their half pints of cider like a last drink before the execution. These chaperoned lunchtime outings to the pub were the only times that Mrs. Andrews now allowed herself to drink. Fearful of losing control, she guarded every porthole to the open seas of her mind.

While her mother napped at home after lunch Maureen walked into the village to do the errands of shopping, the post office, and the cleaners. She stopped at Brown's the bakers and bought a coffee cream cake for her mother's tea and they sat down together a little after four. By the time five o'clock arrived without Doctor Patel Mrs. Andrews was fretting. At five-thirty the phone rang sharply, breaking into their expectant silence. It was Doctor Patel, lost as he never thought he would be, somewhere along the road outside the beech hedge.

"Stay where you are, I am going to walk out into the road to meet you." Maureen left the front door open and walked down the driveway to the beech hedge. Immediately she saw the scruffy car with a neat man on the phone inside.

"Hello Doctor Patel," her voice smiled into the phone and caused him to look up, caught as it were in the headlights of her welcome.

"Hello there." He snapped his phone shut, reaching for his bag and almost sprang out of the car fumbling with his keys and phone and locking the car as he tried to get everything in his left hand to shake Maureen King's extended right one.

"You did find us then, this block is not always easy. Let me show you the way." She turned to walk in front of him down the narrow pathway that led to the front door where Mrs. Andrews was standing, head cocked to one side watching and fixed.

Doctor Patel was surprised at his own quickening heartbeat and eagerness when he saw her and simultaneously breathed in the intoxicating evening air.

"Good evening Mrs. Andrews. I'm Doctor Patel, a consultant psychiatrist for people over sixty-five. I believe you might qualify for my attention." He looked up at the tall, older woman and for a long moment they stared deep into each other's eyes before Mrs. Andrews straightened her back and raised her head once more.

"Don't you count on it," she replied before turning to face the open doorway and leading the way into the house to begin this closing battle. Maureen and Doctor Patel both extended their arms out beckoning the other to follow Mrs. Andrews before Maureen led the way and Doctor Patel followed her. Mrs. Andrews turned to face them when she reached her chair, as if at bay.

"Darling, why don't you sit down? Doctor Patel, would you like this chair? May I get you some tea?"

"Yes please, that would be nice. Thank you." Maureen turned back to her mother.

"Any more for you darling?"

"No thank you, I've had my tea." Her mother was poised between tea and supper, a restless time that always now brought fearful wonderment of imagination and terror. Doctor Patel was waiting for her to sit down into her chair before quietly lowering himself into the matching one by the stairs. He sat still for a moment. Slowly he breathed in the room and the home. He smelt the faint but deep odor of urine that he guessed, correctly, was coming from upstairs and Mrs. Andrews' bedroom.

She absorbed and drank up the modern, urbane smoothness that covered his handsome dark good looks like a stream of fluid silk. She took in his neat navy suit, his blue and white striped shirt with its stiff white collar and red tie. He allowed her this time of watching as an honest hunter is still while their prey searches for danger.

Maureen came back into the room with two mugs of tea and placed one in Doctor Patel's hand while gently setting out a small coaster on the little table beside his chair.

"Thank you." Doctor Patel glanced at Maureen and politely waited until she sat down, perched on the edge of the sofa, across the room. She leant forward holding her mug of tea. All three paused for a moment. Doctor Patel leant forward also, managing to make his posture deferential and not threatening. Mrs. Andrews relaxed back in her chair but her head was cocked and raised. She was smiling now, thrilled at the engagement with the younger man and yet cautious, cautious, as a mouse is mesmerized by a coiled and silent snake.

"Mrs. Andrews, to help me get a better understanding of who you are I am going to ask you a few questions about your life. Please stop me," here Doctor Patel held his hands up palms facing her and waving them from side to side as he repeated, "Please stop me if they are too personal or you do not wish to answer."

He gave another, less benign, pause "for any reason." Maureen sat back on the sofa, trying to relax as a parent would watching their young child's first performance in a school play. She too sensed the danger that was waiting for her mother.

Doctor Patel started slowly with the questions: when and where were you born? Mrs. Andrews answered slowly and correctly. The next few questions were general and allowed her to answer from her current reality. Maureen listened, heart-stoppingly aware of how many lapses of memory her mother was covering with a weak effort of being obtuse and vague.

What Maureen didn't know yet was how aware Doctor Patel was of this also. She watched him follow her mother down the path of her life and it was not until her mother lost her way and took Doctor Patel to a landscape that was not in her mother's reality that Maureen interrupted.

"Do you know the area well?" She spoke quickly in her urgency to head him off from any wrong assumptions he might make about her mother.

"Yes, I live in Hazelbush."

"Do you know the Fernwell Road that now leads to the motorway?"

"Yes," he began but she carried on.

"The big house, Fernwell Hall, with the old rundown garden and the eggs for sale, that is where my mother lived, since she was very young." Maureen added the last hesitantly before continuing. "After my father died she moved to a new house, and then came here closer to the village when she was sixty-four, and has lived here, alone, ever since." Doctor Patel blinked, excited by this connection. He couldn't help himself as he leant forward eagerly.

"I know Fernwell Hall well. Why, we are almost neighbors. I live in The Chestnuts, just two doors away, on the other side of the farm."

Maureen too lent forward, anxious to give him any information, any connection that would cause him to cleave to her mother. She poured out her words quickly in a protective wave with which to shield her mother, to give her a rest from the questions and probings of Doctor Patel's searching.

Doctor Patel listened with interest as Maureen told him the history of his home before catching his eagerness to belong and he pulled himself back to his purpose.

"This is fascinating, I would love to hear more, maybe we can talk about it again." He stood up. Maureen looked at his upright presence and knew a transition was in progress. For a moment his slight, dark, masculine frame was the central point of the room. He moved behind Mrs. Andrews and drew out one of the large mahogany dining room chairs and placed it just behind her, glancing, as he did so, at the heavy needlepoint seat covers. He sat down and propped an elbow on the back of her armchair. She tilted her head back, as if ready to listen to him, but the half smile of her face told Maureen that she was remembering the cradling of a man's arm.

"Now, Mrs. Andrews, I would like—if you will permit me—to ask you some more questions. And I am going to give you three objects to remember. While I ask you the questions I will come back to the objects and ask you to tell them to me again. Would that be all right with you?"

She nodded; how could she refuse? She was too excited to speak and tremulous at the thought of this engagement. He began by giving her three simple objects to remember, two were visible from her chair; a clock and a tree but the third, a dog, was not. He repeated the words, clock, tree, and dog, and she repeated them after him with a hesitant confidence: clock, tree, and dog. Maureen watched as Doctor Patel leant back in the chair like a cat pulling back on its haunches. He asked more seemingly simple questions and encouraged her mother with her nearly, and sometimes even completely, correct answers.

"What day is it? Who is the prime minister? What is your phone number?"

"Can you repeat the three objects I gave you?" Four times he did this and each time the objects became more distant and harder for Mrs. Andrews to recall from the ebbing streams of her memory. She was busy trying to play the question game and dismissed Maureen's fearful look as she had always dismissed Maureen's concerns for her. Doctor Patel gently continued with his questions, repeating some he had asked before but in a different way. "What year were you born? What is the date today?" Why, we could all be hesitant and muddled answering such questions, Maureen thought to herself. But she knew she was searching to buy time for her mother that was not for sale.

At last he was satisfied. Gently, as at the end of a waltz, he let go of Mrs. Andrews' mind with a small bow.

"Thank you very much. You have done very well and been very helpful."

He stood up and put the chair back at the dining room table, noticing again the set of needlepoint chair covers. An industrious and diligent lady, he thought to himself. He did not touch Mrs. Andrews as he turned back to her but said, in a manner she recognized from her own long-ago guardianship of her deceased husband, "I want to have a word with your daughter now and then I will come back and say goodbye to you."

"We can talk in the garden," Maureen broke in. She turned to her mother, "I will bring you some supper, darling, and then we will be back inside." Maureen went into the kitchen and quickly put together a small salad and sandwich. It took no time, this repetitive routine she had done almost every day for over two years.

She returned hoping that the time she had given her mother alone with Doctor Patel had been enough to satisfy her mother and not too long for him. She put the supper tray in front of her mother and ushered Doctor Patel out of the door.

"We will just be outside darling." They went out and around the back of the house into the little garden and sat on the old bench her mother had dragged from home to home. Doctor Patel spoke first.

"You are dealing with dementia of course." His "of course" struck Maureen as swiftly as a French executioner's sword, the cleanness of his strike and professional assessment severed the reality she had been trying to maintain and left it rolling away on the grass in front of them. The trial had been swift, seemingly fair, but the conclusion had been forgone, and she knew it. Before she could utter a word in this new afterlife, he continued.

"We no longer talk about treatment but about management, you understand that?" A statement, a question, a pause? Maureen sat up from her curled position as straight as she could to meet him without actually standing up.

"A vascular dementia," she replied, also a statement and a question.

"Um hum, multifaceted," he acknowledged—and corrected, "of course you want to know how long for: two, three, maybe five years. It depends on the care. I have seen one patient go on for fifteen years. And your mother's heart is strong."

Maureen's own heart sank at the words. Fifteen years of slow erosion. How could her mother bear it, and there would never be enough money for that, three to five years maybe. But she shook herself away from those distant practicalities and returned to Doctor Patel and what he had to say about the here and now.

"She cannot stay here of course—even with what you have put in place she is no longer safe alone. I wonder if she would come to my day hospital? I think not. No, she is too proud a woman. This will come and go you know. Some days will be better than others but always it will continue to get worse. You need to be thinking now of where would be right for her." He paused here, like a doctor giving a diagnosis of terminal cancer. He did not tell her all he knew of the road ahead for her mother; the evaluation based on cold clinical assessment, the nursing homes who put these women to one side, the small wards for the elderly mentally infirm that smell like slowly swirling, blocked toilets. Instead he waited to hear what he knew she had begun to think about. After the diagnosis he could do no more than guide, counsel, prescribe, and to remember, as best he could, the woman he had just met before she disappeared. Sitting on the old bench for a moment he imagined what she must have been like as a young woman living in that old rundown house when both the hall and Mrs. Andrew were young and glorious. He began to go over in his own mind the marks of her personality that he remembered: her flirtatiousness, her effort, the photographs of her family, her pride. He brought himself forward to listen to Maureen.

"I have begun to talk with my mother about Beech Grove. It is just up the road, close enough for her friends to visit. She remembers it as the old hotel it used to be. I have also begun to bring people from Beech Grove's outreach program in three evenings a week and they are getting to know each other. She didn't like it at first but now seems to be accepting it. We go to lunch there once a week together, which she hates. I don't know what else to do. This house is too small for someone else to stay with her all the time, she would drive them crazy and . . ." she paused to draw breath, searching for the next words, "anything might happen."

Doctor Patel nodded his head. Good, he thought, she has already made the decision. Mrs. Andrews would be an appropriate candidate for Beech Grove. She just needed to be encouraged and carry on that path. He sensed Maureen's relief at his assent. Maureen could not think what else to say. She wanted to ask for reassurance that her mother would be all right but knew that all he could give her now would be platitudes. There was no longer any safety.

At that moment Mrs. Andrews appeared from alongside the house. She had only eaten half of her supper, so anxious was she not to let them be alone together for too long. Doctor Patel and Maureen both looked up. Maureen sat, numbed, not wanting this time, where she still might gather some comfort from his words, to end. It was Doctor Patel who was able to smile up at her mother.

"Hello Mrs. Andrews, we were just coming back in."

"Oh yes," Mrs. Andrews tried to make a joke of her words but all three of them felt the fear in her. Doctor Patel rose to his feet. Maureen followed and they both moved towards Mrs. Andrews as she made her way unsteadily on the grass towards them. The sun had dipped down behind the trees that bordered the small communal garden and the first hint of evening cool reminded him he was ready to go home to his supper. Together the three of them walked the short distance back to the door and stood for a moment. Doctor Patel offered his hand first to Mrs. Andrews.

"Goodbye Mrs. Andrews. It has been a pleasure to meet you."

"Goodbye." As Doctor Patel held her hand he felt it tremble like a wounded captured sparrow and he acknowledged, with a slight squeeze of his fingers, that he understood the fear she felt in his presence. He turned to speak to Maureen whose face had lost much of its composure.

"Goodbye, I will be back in touch with Doctor Frank."

"May I call you too?" Maureen spoke quickly, not quite pleading but wanting to make sure there was a doorway open still to him.

"Yes of course, that is no problem. If we need to I can see your mother again. Goodbye."

Maureen put her arm around her mother as Doctor Patel turned on his heel and walked away from the house down the driveway to his car. The two women stood watching as he unlocked the old Honda and climbed in. He turned the car out of the driveway and eased forward into the street. The women stood arm in arm together, waving until he was out of sight.

The Visitor

AFTER LUNCH THE RESIDENTS of Beechnut House returned to their own or the day room for a nap. The staff shifted into an idling second gear of vigilance as they ate their own lunches, slightly larger portions of the gravy and custard-clad two course meal they had just served.

Christmas meant a lot to the residents of Beechnut House. During December, Pam, the administrative nurse in charge of the house, organized a series of Christmas entertainments that filled a ritual memory for her residents. They were touched by the extra kindnesses given and received. The big Christmas party was held at the invitation of the owners, the Simpsons, a mother and son team who showed up once a year to meet the paying children. The owners would not bother Pam again until spring when some fusion of spring cleaning and the Inland Revenue forms on their desks would bring them snooping back, looking to spruce up the place, while spending just enough to give them a tax break for the year.

At 2.30 p.m., Vivian and Patsy began to herd everyone they could into the front parlor room. Chairs were arranged in a semicircle and the dark mahogany upright piano was opened. The black and white keys had been dusted and shone into their ebony glow.

The other residents, the bedridden or the too utterly weary and despondent, stayed in their rooms. Vivian lit the fireplace and the bright flames brought a warm, happy cheer to the otherwise severely dark Victorian room. Joan looked over at Ada who was already getting excited and nervous as she shuffled around the piano stool. She's just showing off, sniffed Joan to herself.

Joan was wearing a blue wool dress along with the pink bead necklace her daughter had given her for her eightieth birthday. Her pearls, like most of her rings, had been discreetly put away for safe keeping. But daily she wore her wedding ring, a gold bracelet from her lover, and this necklace from her daughter.

Neil Parker, the accordionist, stood at the back of the room. He was talking to Vivian who was busy helping everyone to their seats. Neil liked to come to the old people's home over Christmas. During these visits he made up for his working life as a not very honest or successful car salesman. Now in his mid-sixties he is aware enough to be grateful for the gift of music he still enjoys. He is a tall, trim man, but with a closed, half-hearted smile. The good looks of his youth had made him lazy. He had counted on his body to sell cars to the husbands of needy housewives, guilty at their neglect of their worn women. He looked at these women getting seated around him and smiled. He believes in his role of a seasoned seducer. He has no thought that he will ever be one of them.

※❀❀❀⁂

Joan's posture is still good and she always sits up very straight in her chair. Despite a hip operation for arthritis three years ago she has lost very little height. She is a tall woman, now thinning with oncoming death. She moves her head slowly back and forth as if watching a tennis match, while Vivian guides in the late comers from their afternoon toilet. Though time flows past her through the days, she sniffs disapprovingly at their tardiness. She knows that on waking there will be breakfast. Then it is time to dress and wait for a visitor. Most mornings one of her old friends drops in for a coffee as they go to town to shop. On entering Beechnut House, unknowingly she has switched her place in her remaining friends' engagement diaries. Two friends drop her immediately, claiming not their fear, but their own infirmities as enough reason not to visit her. Others have placed her on their duty roster to be seen biweekly with loyalty. Only one friend, Heather, visits her weekly, loving her as friends need to be loved, for fellowship's sake. Joan never looked with expectation to these visits but accepted them as they happened. Memories float as remembered dreams through her days and nights as her friends try to take her back into her life or forward into theirs. She likes it when they help her with her lunch tray or going to the bathroom. Best of all is when they just sit with her. She doesn't even mind the television that is now a bother and a confusion for her. She never watches it alone for herself. But it is no longer a rude intrusion to have it on when someone visits with her. It is almost comforting. She becomes a hostess again, giving them a distraction in the television as she had with her company in her home.

After lunch her daughter came to visit for the afternoon. Louise brought her knitting and they sat together quietly through tea time. Finally her daughter was accepting of the role she has trained her for, that of handmaiden. Joan only had to shift her position and Louise would look up, be ready to pour another cup of tea or take her to the bathroom. Sometimes Louise would sort and tidy the hanging clothes in the closet; the ones that did not belong to her mother she returned discreetly to the laundry room. It was soothing for Joan to see her daughter knit. She was convinced that the math of counting, making or following patterns had helped her hold onto her mind for as long as she had.

But when it struck she had known. That day, this she could remember. Heather and John, her husband, had stopped by to bring her weekly eggs. She remembered it had also been Christmas time then, but how many years ago? She had been shaking all morning, feeling her heart beating harder and faster, harder and faster. The sound of the door bell had jolted her so that she almost fell down from its sharp ring. She had managed to let them in and then, then what happened? She could remember the doctor coming to the house, some fuss and him saying she must go to the hospital. An ambulance. She had been fearful and out of control, afraid of the looming Santa Clauses and gnomes placed as Christmas decorations around the wards. She could remember. She was sure. But why go back to harsh memories? Now was enough.

Joan sat in her chair, waiting through her memories for everyone to be seated and for Neil and Ada to begin the music.

Neil began with "Away in a Manger." Everyone knew the words and now understood that this was to be an afternoon of carol singing. Two of the ladies were mouthing the words with a masticating motion, as if the music were their food. Open sing, open chew, what was the difference thought

Joan, and she sat with her mouth firmly closed and her hands folded primly in her lap.

The first carol ended. Neil gave Ada a nod and she dropped her hands into the bouncing opening chords of "Ding Dong Merrily on High." But still the ladies sat quietly, though Elizabeth in her wheelchair in the corner had joined the singing, moving her hands to conduct Neil from her lap.

"Come on ladies. You all know this one," pleaded Vivian again. Her legs ached and there was still the tea trolley to get out at three-thirty.

At three-fifteen the door bell rang with an abrupt, masculine force. All the ladies heard it. The door was opened and closed loudly, feet were stamped on the door mat, a wet mackintosh could be heard to be peeled off and an umbrella thumped and shaken into the hall stand. So it was raining outside after all, thought Joan.

The ladies waited, their attention even less on Neil's music than before. Hope for a visitor never left them. Though for most of the ladies it was hard, even for half an hour, to pull themselves into a present and actual reality. Their engagement with the world they had slowly slid from was something to which they only dreamt of returning. Memory was light in their heads and did not linger.

Meanwhile they listened, knowing the sequence of sounds that would come from the hallway. A quiet silence as the visitor signed the guest book. They could have been entering a giant corporate office in the capital rather than a small country home for the elderly and infirm. The staff were supposed to review the book weekly, to check who had visitors, who did not and what, if anything, to do about it.

The ladies waited for the book signing to be over. If it was a male visitor, and the ladies all knew it was, one of the staff, also hungry for testosterone, might waylay and hold him to themselves. The visitor might only have an hour and a half and begin that clock ticking from when they turned off the car engine. Occasionally there would be the visitor who had surrendered this time and had no agenda other than being in the presence of their beloved.

After the conversation with a staff member there were footsteps, upstairs to see Margaret or Peggy or towards the day room where Betty and Jill sat forever, or maybe today, for a special visit, into the front parlor.

The voices in the hallway of Patsy and the visitor made Joan sit up even straighter. Neil and Ada continued playing, moving onto "O Little Town of Bethlehem, How still we see thee lie," but Joan wasn't hearing them any more. She knew that voice. Had known it since it was but a baby's cry, then a pip squeaking soprano, listened attentively until it had settled into the rich baritone of its maturity and left home. She saw Michael step through the doorway into the front parlor and look for her. She waited for his smile which came as soon as he saw her. She watched closely for any look of surprise, or disgust that so often crossed the face of the first time visitors when they came to see her here. But Michael's face beamed in happy recognition.

"Hello Aunt Joan. Great to see you. Merry Christmas." He handed her the box of chocolates he had brought from the new shop in town. He reached down to kiss her and take in his the hand she raised to welcome him.

Quickly Vivian pulled over a chair from the back of the room and placed it beside Joan. Imploring him with this gesture to stay and by his presence help lift the stagnant energy in the room.

Neil and Ada had stopped playing. Neil pulled the strap of his accordion over his head and laid the instrument down on the long dining table behind him. Ada returned to the circle of women, not wanting to miss a biscuit with her tea.

"Tea trolley's here," Patsy called out as she wheeled the trolley into the parlor. The relief of this ritual was palpable. It was as if a bell had been rung and a difficult class come to an end. Vivian checked around for the usual suspects who would need another bathroom visit before taking in a cup of tea.

"Joan do you need the toilet?" Vivian asked in too loud a voice.

"No thank you," Joan replied primly, pretending shock at this intrusion, embarrassed at being asked in front of Michael. To her relief Michael was looking at her with a conspiratorial grin.

"Ready for tea Aunt Joan?" he asked, as Patsy turned to Michael. She liked him, Joan could tell.

Joan looked at Michael over her cup of tea. He called her Aunt Joan. So this must be the boy she thought. But she was remembering him, Michael's father Christopher. The same height, the same breadth, the same black turned grizzled gray hair and the same hands, big and sturdy but gentle.

Joan tried to pay attention. Michael was telling her about the family. His wife, Jill, had a new job. The two boys had almost, once again, left home. He laughed when he told her this, how many of his friends' children also never quite seemed to get going after finishing university and leave as his generation had.

Joan nodded and added, "I know what you mean," as if she did. Last year she would have known. Would have remembered stories that her friends would have also told her.

Tea was over quickly. Patsy went once around with the trolley and then began collecting tea plates and cups and saucers, napkins, and crumbs and Vivian was doing another toilet round.

Neil, glad to be rid of his tepid tea, asked Roderick, the only male resident, to join him at the piano for a last half hour of tunes. Roderick got up and pushed his chair back roughly. He shuffled behind Elizabeth in her wheelchair and sat down on the piano stool. Neil slung the accordion strap back over his shoulder and was about to ripple through another Christmas carol when Roderick brought both hands down hard on the piano keys and into "Let's Do It," an old Cole Porter melody. A shudder fluttered around the room. Here was a song of the deep past, fixed in youthful memory. The ladies shifted in their chairs. Joan raised her head, her eyes darting from side to side, searching, and softly began to sing the words. Neil smiled as his hands roamed the smooth keys of his instrument. He too liked these old songs. There was a comfort in them, a surety of love that had been, that existed. Roderick's own memories had taken him over and he swung easily into another melody. Neil followed along, glad for a change not to be leading. He smiled directly at Joan and her visitor. They were enjoying the music. Michael looked up and smiled back; both men knew how little it took to satisfy lonely women.

Michael turned back to his Aunt Joan and gently taking one of her hands in his leant over her and whispered, "Care to dance Aunt Joan?" She looked up at him. A remembered move drew her to her feet and into his arms. He guided her into the center of the small circle of chairs. His arm enclosed her thin waist. She is so frail he must be careful not to crush her. Joan's arms reached up towards his neck. She moved to the music and to memory. Slowly she leant in closer until her head curled onto his chest. She trembled with the thrill of it. Inhaled the smell of him, the damp wool jacket that carried the odors of a man's drinking bar. The softness of the warm, viyella shirt next to his skin sank her into the heaven of his father's embrace.

The embraces of her sister's husband, the one she had loved longer and deeper than her own. But, that but, that had kept the beat of their passion alive for over the thirty years of dual ownership. The years of loneliness, loss and anguish hid from her now. All she felt was a trembling desire to remain held in these strong arms and to drink in the perfume of his masculine tenderness.

Michael found himself humming in her ear as he gently rocked her from side to side, moving her in tiny steps around their improvised dance floor. Roderick and Neil played on, following with "So in Love with You." The ladies sat quietly, also rocking from side to side. They too were lost in their own memories. Even Vivian, her elbows rested on the back of Elizabeth's wheelchair, her tired legs forgotten, enjoyed as much as waited through this moment.

Michael held his Aunt Joan carefully until the tune came to an end. Slowly his arm slipped from around her waist as he released her. He took her hand, which lay still in his. He looked down at her sad yet smiling face and said, "Thank you Aunt Joan. That was lovely."

She nodded and let him lead her back to her chair.

The Dentist

THE SUN SHONE ON Margaret's head and through her fine white hair, giving her an unruly, angelic halo. She sat in her big wing-backed chair finishing her breakfast. Her porridge was long gone. Now she dips leggings of brown bread into the boiled egg shell and scoops up the last of the egg yolk, staining her lips yellow. When Jeanie came into the room to say "Good morning," Margaret looked up with a smile, and knows this meant they will be together for the day.

"Will you be ready for me in half an hour Margaret?" Jeanie smiles down at the woman sitting in the chair.

"Yes please," Margaret mumbles. Neither of them notices her soft words. They are part of the daily dialogue the two women easily settled into over the months since Margaret first came to The Hall. Margaret likes the way Jeanie gives her time to catch up with the morning yet appreciates how efficiently she gets things done. In Jeanie's presence Margaret knows she will not slip or fall. That alone helped her to adjust and accept her room, number 4, at The Hall.

Twenty minutes later Jeanie returned to take the breakfast tray away.

"It looks like you enjoyed that," she said with another smile, taking the egg-covered spoon out of the tea cup and and putting it back on the saucer. "Ready for a wash now?"

"Yes. I think so." Margaret got up out of her chair and gathered her dressing gown around her body. She walked to the bathroom to begin her lifelong routine of morning ablutions.

Like many women of Margaret's generation, who married military officers, Margaret had all of her teeth extracted before they were stationed overseas. The acquisition of two sets of dentures was as an important rite of passage as a string of pearls on her twenty-first birthday. For people with perpetual bleeding gums, rotting teeth or even a demanding pregnancy, it was also common for dentists to take out a complete set of teeth for no other reason than it would be "easier in the long run." For this generation of women "the long run" stretched out ahead to sixty plus years of dentures. The family dentist, Mr. Roe, suggested, as he did to all his patients, that Margaret have two sets of dentures. He instructed her to change her teeth every day so that both sets would remain pliable and comfortable in her mouth though, he said, one set would always be more comfortable than the other. Don't ask me why that is, he added. And so, from when she was twenty-five, to her eighty-eighth year, Margaret had always had two sets of dentures and changed them each and every day.

Margaret's husband Edward had been posted to Ceylon for five years. She had enjoyed their time together there. She became used to the staff, even the ayah who, when her son Simon was born, came and took him from her. But she had insisted on nursing her son. Sometimes, while watching his gumming mouth pull on her breasts, she had run her tongue around her own mouth, wondering what she might be missing along with her teeth.

Jeanie and Margaret moved in the rhythms of working in and with service throughout their separate lives. Now they have come together and are each glad of the other. Jeanie finished making the bed and laid out fresh clothes for Margaret. When new residents arrive they are supposed to be able to make these choices and dress themselves. But slowly capacity erodes, and staff expectations and encouragement give way to haste. The residents lose drive and accommodations are made on both sides. Jeanie goes to the bathroom, smiling at Margaret, standing in front of the washbasin, stark naked, but for her wedding ring and blue slippers. Her now slim bottom droops over veined legs while her sagging pale breasts hold only the faintest memory of her taut virginal innocence. Margaret smiled too. Margaret knew it was safe to share with Jeanie that she had forgotten, for the moment, what it is she should be doing next.

"Look at you Margaret. Are you washed?" Margaret nodded and smiled some more.

"Fanny done?" Margaret grinned back at her. "Here, let me finish you up." Jeanie moved forward to Margaret and deftly attended to those private creases that hide crumbs, wadded paper and dry, flaking skin. She powdered Margaret's body gently, taking talc under the light breasts and down through her buttock creases.

"If you sit down I can do your toes." Margaret sat down on the laundry stool that she had brought from home to home since she was a girl. Jeanie knelt in front of her and prying the frozen curled toes apart she smoothed powder between them.

"Now you are all set. Except for your teeth. Which set is it?" They laughed together while Jeanie rose from her knees and returned to the sink. She reached up to the shelf. She felt the warmth of the blue pot as fresh and so opened the pink one but found only one bottom plate resting in the denture liquid. Her heart sank.

"What happened to your teeth Margaret? There is only the bottoms here." Margaret looked up, startled, and tried to stand too quickly. She almost fell but held the towel rail to steady herself.

Deftly Jeanie popped the same but now cleaned dentures into Margaret's mouth and hurried her across the hallway back to Margaret's room. With Jeanie's help Margaret dressed in a skirt, blouse, and cardigan. On went the long support stockings but Margaret refused to put on her shoes and stayed in her slippers. She was subdued as she went with Jeanie downstairs to the sitting room.

The weather outside was vile. The rain pelted down on the long glass windows which, on days like this, brought the blank paleness of a gray sky threateningly close. Though the fire was on and the room was warm, the ladies felt the cold. They shivered against the weather, fearing its memory.

The front door banged shut, there was the stamping of feet and shaking of an umbrella. Someone had arrived and Jeanie went to meet them.

"Hello Simon. How is the weather out there?"

"Cold and wet. How is the world in here, Jeanie? How's mother?"

"In a bit of a fuss I think. We couldn't find her top plate this morning. It must have fallen out last night. The girls are going through the laundry now. So far we haven't been able to track it down. But we will." She smiled brightly at him. "Don't worry. We'll find them. Go in and see her. She's in the morning room. You are just in time for a coffee." Simon had retired from his engineering firm three years ago. He had chosen The Hall for Margaret as being convenient for him and his family. Almost every day he walked through the village to visit her but on days like this one he drove the old Escort car over. He entered the morning room as Denise was about to serve Margaret her coffee.

"Ah. You're here." Margaret had been watching the door, waiting for Simon to arrive and help her.

"Good morning Mother. How are you today?" He bent down to give her a kiss which she dismissed.

"They've lost my teeth," she replied.

"Thank you Denise." Simon held the mug of weak, warm coffee that Denise handed him. "I'm sure they will show up," he continued.

"I will need a new pair," she said firmly.

"Hang on Mother," Simon half laughed and almost spilt his coffee. "They will show up. I bet they are behind your bed or wrapped up in a sheet somewhere."

"Jeanie's already looked. They are probably in the rubbish. Gone. I must have my teeth." Simon suppressed a sigh.

"Let them have a good look mother. They really might show up."

"I need my teeth." Mother and son pressed their lips together in unison as if to prevent any more teeth from escaping. Simon left as lunch was being served. He spoke with Jeanie on his way out.

"Any sign of the teeth?" he asked. She gave a half smile and shook her head.

"We'll keep looking. I'm sure we'll find them." Both of them knew that the longer the teeth went missing the harder it would be to retrieve them. By now they could be shaken out of a sheet, into the trash or crushed in the laundry. Almost a worse fate was that they would be returned to another resident who would not notice the mistake. It would be an unsuspecting mortician who would have the final manipulation of ill fitting dentures to deal with.

Margaret did not sleep well that night. She kept waking, clucking her mouth together checking that both plates were still in place. The next day she became more agitated with the conscious knowledge that she was taking out, washing and putting back into her mouth the same set of teeth. She dressed but stayed in her room for morning coffee and returned to her room directly after lunch. Simon found her there when he arrived to visit at tea time.

"Hello Mother," he said as he always did. "How are you today?"

Margaret didn't reply. She cast a quick glance at him before turning her head back to the unused tea tray in front of her. Jeanie has seen Simon come in and arrived with a mug of tea for him too.

"Hello Simon," she said brightly as she handed him the mug.

"Hello Jeanie. Any luck?" He left the question open, so as not to say the word—teeth. She shook her head and gave a pointed look in Margaret's direction. Simon shrugged. He was not going to make the missing dentures as big an issue as his mother seemed to be doing.

Margaret stayed in her room the following day and the next day Jeanie found her lying on her bed as if for an afternoon nap. It was as if now she believed that they had taken her teeth from her. The whole rhythm of her life was disrupted. Finally in exasperation Simon exclaimed, "You don't need another set of dentures Mother. It is not as if you are going anywhere."

"I do need them," she replied firmly. And with this exchange the value of the remaining time left to her and to him lay between them. Would it be years? He couldn't see that, maybe more than a year but not stretching into two. As Simon watched his mother he realized that they were marking her remaining days on different calendars. He was crossing off days, easing himself towards an acceptance of her approaching death. For Margaret each day still held a promise, if not of an adventure the possibility of being lived through, and was marked in her mind with a check on its completion.

"Life is very precious," Margaret said one day. The day's journey was still an accomplishment, an achievement, a winning of the battle of her ebbing strength and the eventual collapse of her body. Two days later, when Simon came for coffee he found Margaret still in bed.

"Hello Mother. Not up yet? Jeanie not on duty today?" Margaret was usually one of the first residents dressed. Simon looked at his mother for a long moment before reaching into her bedside locker and pulling out the old telephone directory that they had brought with her from her home to The Hall.

"Just in case we need it," Margaret had said when he had tried to throw it out instead of packing it for her move. Simon thumbed through the Ds to dentists until he read, "Denture and bridge repair. We make house calls." He picked up the phone and dialed the number. Doctor Scott's receptionist wasn't at all surprised by Simon's request.

"Yes, of course. These things happen more often than you would think. And they," she herded everyone over seventy together in the phrase, "they do miss their dentures you know." She finished brightly. "Your mother is at The Hall. Just the uppers you say. Doctor Scott can come over tomorrow afternoon. He will need to make an impression of course. Can your mother sit still? Good. It will be five working days after the impression so let's see, tomorrow is Wednesday, they could be ready by the following Wednesday, possibly even Tuesday. That will be four hundred pounds payable on receipt of the dentures." Simon found himself agreeing even as he thought, my God four hundred pounds, if she lives four months that is a hundred pounds a month, for a half set of teeth. He sighed. How long had it been since he had done something for her that she actually wanted? He was measuring the worth of his mother's comfort, his mother' desires, against the value of her money and he knew it.

The next day Margaret got out of bed, dressed and sat in her chair, waiting. Her mind was fixed on the coming appointment. Simon waited with her. It was after lunch before Doctor Scott announced his arrival with a firm knock on the half open door to Margaret's room. Doctor Scott wore a short white lab coat. In a hospital setting he looked like a laboratory technician but in the homes of the elderly he served he had long ago realized that a short coat was more reassuring than intimidating. He carried a small plastic toolbox that, apart from its green color, looked remarkably similar to the toolbox Mr. Robson would bring when he had come to the house and dealt with the plumbing fluctuations of Margaret's kitchen and bathroom.

"Come in, come in," said Simon, reaching forward to pull the door farther open. "I'm Simon Fitzpatrick. This is my mother, Margaret Fitzpatrick. Mother," he called too loudly and cheerfully, "this is Doctor Scott, the dentist. He has come to make you a new denture."

Margaret raised her hand in a half wave welcome.

Doctor Scott nodded and spoke briefly to Simon but looked at Margaret in her chair whom he had come to attend. He took in the faded chintz fabric encasing her upright stick figure. Today she was dressed in a dark red wool pleated skirt with a matching light top that covered a warm blue-flowered blouse. The blouse and the chair cover were of the same era of floral overflow. They lay beside each other, too old for competition. Her slippered feet softly rested on the carpet.

Simon stood back as Doctor Scott crossed the small room towards Margaret and bent forward to introduce himself. He leaned down, coming close to Margaret and spoke, just to her.

"Hello Mrs. Fitzpatrick. I'm Doctor Scott. I've come to see about your dentures." Margaret, whose eyes had been shut as if in a trance, blinked them open again and looked at him. She did not find his presence too close.

"Hello," she said.

"May I sit down?" he asked. She nodded and waved her hand, this time in a royal command to signal, of course. Simon pushed the only other chair in the room forward before retreating to sit on the bed. Doctor Scott sat and looked at Margaret who, with her hands now folded tamely in her lap, returned his gaze.

"I understand you need an upper plate replaced."

Margaret nodded.

"I can do that for you. I'll need to take an impression of your mouth. You will have to sit very still. Can you do that?" His question was that of a gym coach, explaining a new maneuver to an eager student. A small smile crossed Margaret's face and she nodded again.

"All right. I'll get my things ready. No need for you to get up." Margaret was trying to rise out of the chair as if they were going somewhere together. "Unless you need to?" Doctor Scott inquired politely. She shook her head.

Doctor Scott rose from the chair and opened his toolbox, carefully laying the implements of his trade out on the tray table beside Margaret.

"The bathroom?" he asked. Simon sprung up off the bed to show him the way. He disappeared. Simon looked at Margaret and smiled. He almost said something cheerful but Margaret silenced him with a look.

Doctor Scott returned to Margaret's room with a small plastic bowl of warm water and a towel. He helped her remove the dentures and rinse her mouth. She followed his lead wordlessly. Doctor Scott wiped her lips gently and then turned back to the tray table. Deftly, with unhurried movements he mixed up the pink goop and scraped it from the bowl into the mold. He leaned forward and, with one hand, applied a little pressure on Margaret's chin and said softly, "Now open." As she did so he slipped the mold into her mouth and pressed it firmly up to her palate, at the same time easing himself back down onto the chair in front of her. They sat so, together in silence, for a full minute. As the pressure became more intense Margaret struggled not to gag. She tried to move but could not. She raised her hand searching for relief. Doctor Scott reached out with his free hand and holding hers gently returned it to her lap. Their hands lay woven together among her skirt's red wool pleats for the four more minutes needed for the mold to set. From his seat on the bed Simon watched his mother relax, be comforted and made whole once more.

The Letter M

AT TEN FORTY-FIVE IN the morning the hearse pulled up to the steps of Saint Mark's Church on the Marylebone Road. The coffin lay silently waiting, covered in three tasteful wreaths: two of lilies from his club and solicitor partners and one of red and white roses from his wife and two daughters. Not that anyone expected the coffin to be anything but silent but there was always the question, randomly escaping from somebody's mind, as they climb the steps to the church door. Does someone at the mortuary stay with the body all through the final night-time shift to make sure the soul of the deceased had truly departed? These questions passed through more than one mind of the friends and family of Derrick Bradshaw as they climbed the steps of Saint Mark's Church that cold Tuesday morning in March. The hearse was early, as is befitting, but never guaranteed. Morticians and their charges, unlike some brides on their wedding days, like to be seen to be on time. The mortuary attendants were smartly dressed in their morning suits and stood to attention on the church steps. Their gloved hands were clasped in front of their bodies and they bowed from the waist down in a silent greeting to each of the incoming mourners. The waiting family and friends mingled with solemnity and respectful quiet. There would be ample opportunity for catching up on the goings-on of each other's families later, at the post service gathering that now had become part of the modern day memorial for the dead.

"Please join us for refreshments and further celebration of Derrick's life and work at the Club . . ." was printed in the order of service and with the service beginning at 11 a.m. most people were expecting hearty club sandwiches for lunch.

Moyra was not expecting anything. She didn't know how she could be, seeing his wife and family sitting so close to the coffin. Elizabeth, unknowing of her existence, the daughters finally aware of her, but how much aware she still didn't know. Yet she wanted to linger, to hold what she could of Derrick still in her physical presence.

Moyra was absorbed within the friends and relations now arriving at the church. The immediate family were already gathered, sequestered away in the waiting room designated for "before." There was another room for "after," and it was the church warden's responsibility to make sure that the groups did not get confused.

Derrick's wife Elizabeth and her two daughters, Allison and Linda, were each dressed in black. In the waiting room Elizabeth sank into a chair, suddenly too weary after the last few months to stand more than she must. Allison and Linda, both with a more practical bent and sterner outlook, stood and looked to see how the order of service had turned out. It is good, thought Allison, we got it all in there and it looks nice. Linda looked at the photographs of her father that they had chosen. On the front was one she had taken two years ago, before the illness had taken hold of him and begun its voracious meal of his body. On the back was one of Derrick as a young university student, looking a little silly, a little cocky, hamming it up in his tweed jacket and with his University of London scarf wrapped around his neck, protecting him. From what, she wondered, was it the London smog of the fifties or just the country cold air of a winter break? Whichever, he was smiling, hopelessly optimistic, as all of that generation were. He had completed his national service in the navy, and was half way through university and his law degree. Derrick became a successful barrister, Queen's Counsel, and had little cause to worry or to stray from the marked path of his life. And yet he had, thought Linda, and wondered again about the phone call and the woman behind the voice of Moyra O'Sullivan whom she had spoken to just four days before.

It had been Allison who had found the name Moyra O'Sullivan in their father's address book when they sat down in his study on the afternoon of his death. He had died as he had lived, conveniently for others, at nine-thirty in the morning, allowing for the doctor's visit and removal of his body to take place before the family returned home to a light luncheon of Scotch broth soup, laced with a glass of sherry. Elizabeth was finally too weak to drink the sherry straight. The last two weeks of Derrick's illness had been hard on them all. Settled into a hospice home waiting for death to take its turn had seemed like a good idea at the time but the hospice had been a long hour's drive from their home. Derrick was made comfortable. The daughters were both grateful. During the first year the illness had progressed slowly. But over the last few months it gained momentum and encroached on him faster than he could stave it off. The shots fired into him dulled his pain, then his senses, until the flame of his wick, with a final sputter, had surrendered its light. Allison and Linda watched their father slip away and their mother flounder in a fog of "calming medicines" which for the first time they came to realize had been her companion for several years. It had been an exhausting time for these two competent women. After lunch Linda took Elizabeth upstairs and tucked her into bed with a hot water-bottle. Allison went to the study and began to go through their father's small, worn leather address book. She made a list of relatives to call. It was ever thus with these two, Linda the Mary to Allison's Martha. They had made good wives and mothers with both those traits and over the last couple of years managed to serve their parents well. Both knew that now would come long shifts of caring and responsibility for their mother.

Linda made two cups of instant Nescafe coffee and brought them up to the study, placing one in front of Allison who was sitting at her father's old roll top desk. They had known this desk since childhood. Over the last weeks they had come here, sticking their heads around the door and still expected to see him sitting in his chair, turn around, look down through his bifocal glasses at them and smile. He had always smiled at them when they came in. Not once, as tiny children, teenagers drifting through with unasked questions, as young women with "things to tell him" or later even with things to remind him of, had he made them feel that their interruptions were anything other than a delight to his life.

Now they sat in his study alone, Allison on the leather swivel-chair and Linda in the old cozy chintz-covered chair.

"Where do we start?" asked Linda.

"Uncle Jimmy, I suppose, and then let him tell the cousins. We should let them know before the papers and arrangements, don't you think?"

"Oh yes. We can always say what we think it will be and then they can look for it in *The Times* or *The Telegraph*. Shall we finish that this afternoon?" The girls had already begun the notice for the papers. It was just a matter of the details. "No flowers by request. Donations to your local Hospice or the Macmillan Foundation."

"And Uncle Richard, we should let him know."

"Yes, he can tell the firm and then that's done."

"Yes. That's good. Who else have you got?"

"The usual, the city and golf club secretaries, their bridge group. Does Mummy want to call anyone?" Linda shrugged.

"Mummy should call Aunt Mary, she is her sister after all. But I don't know if she will be able to." Her voice softened. The sisters looked at each other before both taking refuge in staring out of the window for a long moment.

"All right. Let me see who else there is in here that we might have missed. Do we have to go through the whole Christmas card list or can we let most of them pick it up in the papers?"

"I think I'll start with Daddy's address book and see what is in there."

"Right. Want more coffee?"

"I'm fine thanks." And with that both women set about their tasks. Allison opened the address book and began writing out a list of names and telephone numbers on a separate piece of paper. All were familiar to her from one part of her father's work or parents' social world. Except when Allison turned the page to O. She came across an entry she didn't recognize, Moyra O'S, and a phone number. Her father's handwriting, neat at the best of times, seemed to have been particularly careful with this entry. She couldn't tell exactly how but there was something measured about the letters on the page. Linda was in the kitchen setting up a tea-tray for later when Allison came downstairs with the phone book in her hand.

"Any idea who this is?" she asked.

"Who what is?" Linda was struggling with her mother's old cake tin, trying to pry the lid off.

"This Moyra O'S. Here, look." Allison showed her the entry in the phone book.

"No idea. Should we ask Mummy?" and then as the same thought crossed their minds they looked at each other and Linda continued, "Maybe not." A silence sat in the kitchen with them as they both looked at the book and thought about their father. About his quietness, his resigned loneliness as he patiently dealt with his wife's increasingly neurotic behavior that had left the girls impatient and saddened at the lives of their parents. With a slight smile Linda asked, "Do you think we should phone her?"

Allison too began to smile. "Maybe we should. She might be someone who would want to know."

"Well I certainly want to know. Let's phone her now." And Linda put down the stubborn teacake tin and followed her sister back up to their father's study. Allison sat down at her father's desk once more and paused before she picked up the phone.

"I wonder," she said, "I wonder if there is anything in his diary?" She reached into the top drawer where Derrick had put his keys, a pen knife, and his small engagement diary as he had undressed to climb into bed the weeks before he had died. For the last few weeks the pages were almost blank. There were a few notations of long standing but they were engagements he had not kept and neither, to the girls' memory, had their mother. Derrick had also an old habit of jotting down what he had done during the day. A word, garden, a number after the names Philip and Michael would be his golf score of that day. Allison turned the pages backwards to the week before Christmas when the entries, written now in a visibly frail hand, had stopped. But there on December 18th was a small M in the corner of that date's space. She turned the page back again, slowly, the 15th, 12th, 6th and on and on back into the last year of his life two or three times on the week's page Derrick had written the letter M.

"Look at this." Allison showed her sister the diary. "It goes all the way through the year."

"Oh my God. Do you think it is her?" Linda responded more excited than shocked. "Where are his old diaries?" Two pairs of hands reached into the second drawer down from the top on the right-hand side of his desk. An old rubber band held the last five years together and an even older rubber band the previous five. The girls took out the previous year and began going through it. There it was, the letter M, bolder then as Derrick's health had been. It seemed regularly placed, twice a week, occasionally three times, and very occasionally only once, but going back through two, three books it seemed that M had been a regular date for Derrick. It took two further diaries to come to the first M entry. There it was: Moyra O'Sullivan and a phone number. A week later was another more complete entry: Moyra and an address, 39 Queen Street, Primrose Hill.

"That must be her. My God four, no five years and we had no idea."

"What shall we do?" Allison asked. "She must have known about us, about Daddy's illness."

"Yes of course she must. And we should let her know about today, and also somehow that we know about her too. No wonder he was able to be so patient with Mummy."

"Yes. That would be it. Poor Mummy, do you think she has any idea?"

"I don't know. What do we do about that?"

"Well I don't think we should ask her, do you? Mummy do you know if Daddy had a lady friend?" And for the first time in weeks the sisters were overtaken by childhood silly giggles. Finally Linda stopped laughing enough to say, "Why don't we call, now. If she is someone special for Daddy," and she smiled at the thought before becoming serious again, "then she'd want to know." Linda stood forward, leaning over the back of her father's old chair.

"Yes, you're right. I'll do it now." And holding the old diary of five years ago open to the first entry for Moyra O'Sullivan, Allison dialed the number.

<hr />

Moyra picked up the phone after the second ring. The last two months had been filled with a lonely sadness for her as she waited, reading the daily papers from back to front looking to see if what she knew was in store for Derrick had come to pass. On Derrick's last visit they had sat by the window looking over her little terrace garden. The nesting tables between them held a small bowl of uneaten nuts. Even the homemade lemonade served in a cut-glass Pimm's jug instead of their usual sherry now lay untouched. He had become weaker by the day, and she saw it every time he climbed the stairs to her flat. She knew what the disease and the treatment were doing to him.

"I don't know how much longer I can go on," Derrick had said to her that day.

"You are being so brave darling. If ever," she caught her breath not "when" she thought, not "when," "if ever this becomes too much you know I'll understand, don't you?" A silence hovered over the still-full jug of lemonade and the bowl of nuts.

Derrick reached out his hand to hers across the little nesting tables and began to speak.

"Do you know the story about Alexander the Great?"

"What's that?" she asked with a smile.

"When Alexander the Great lay on his deathbed he had three last wishes. The first wish was that his coffin be carried on the shoulders of the most eminent physicians of his realm so that people would know that the doctors did not have, in the face of death, the power to heal." Derrick finished and looked across to Moyra. She didn't ask about the other two wishes. Instead she squeezed his hand and said, "You will phone when you can, I know." Derrick nodded.

"Yes, of course," he replied, and added, "I'm so sorry." They sat in silence watching the afternoon light begin to fade. As dusk crept close, Derrick sighed and stood up.

"It is time I was going." They embraced tenderly, holding each other for a long time. This was the moment of their physical goodbye. Now he would return to the habit of his family and draw it around him as a nun would against the cold.

As Derrick crossed the street he looked back up once more, seeing Moyra watch him from the window as she had every time he had come to be with her. Then he turned the corner and hailed a taxi that would let him out one street away from his home.

Derrick managed to get to his study every day. Elizabeth never bothered him there, and he was careful to phone when one of the girls was not expected to visit. Now one or other of his daughters came to the house every day. He smiled, sure they had worked out a schedule between them. The family roles were reversed. Their daughters talked about him and Elizabeth as they had about the girls, when they were young. When they were young, he thought. That had been a long time ago. Derrick phoned Moyra daily up until the last three weeks when the silence between them stretched along the river that wound through the city and separated their homes.

The ring of the telephone broke the silence that now surrounded Moyra. She was sitting next to the nesting tables that held her copy of *The Telegraph* and her reading glasses. The afternoon sunlight was dim, and she cherished this moment and the memory it brought her of Derrick's last visit.

"Hello." Moyra's voice was quiet, unemotional.

"Hello, is this Moyra O'Sullivan?"

"Yes, speaking."

"Oh, hello." Allison's voice was tentative, more hesitant than she had hoped it would be. "This is Allison Wright. I'm Derrick Bradshaw's daughter, one of them, I have a sister, Linda."

"Yes," Moyra broke in quickly. Her body already knowing what her mind had not received. "Yes," she said again.

"I believe you knew my father." Unnecessary, thought Allison, unnecessary, of course this is her. "I'm afraid I have sad news. My father," her voice broke as she suddenly realized that this was the first phone call she had made, even before Uncle Jimmy. She continued, "My father died this morning." She paused, wondering what to say next. "I think he was quite comfortable at the end. I'm so sorry." There was a long pause as Moyra took in the words and tried to reshuffle them into something like, "He's quite comfortable now." But it didn't work.

"Thank you. Thank you for letting me know," she said. And then stupidly, but essential for her, she asked, "Where is he?" Allison drew in her breath, taking in that the woman on the other end of the line still yearned for their father.

"He's at Buckingham's. We have him at Buckingham's." A wave of kindness pushed Allison to continue, "I expect if you called ahead you could visit. Mornings might be best." Both women understood that it would be afternoon and evening times before those friends and family, for whom a visitation to the deceased was an important part of grieving, would call. "We haven't made the final arrangements yet. It will be in the papers when we do." And then another soft afterthought as her words fell on the loving, sad silence from the telephone line, "Would you like me to phone when we have made the arrangements?"

"Thank you," said Moyra. "If that wouldn't be too much trouble."

"Not at all. I'm so sorry." Allison paused again. Sorry to be the messenger, sorry for the end of something she had only just discovered, that their father had found a place of happiness and peace, beyond the confines of his male-dominated club and office. "I'll phone when I have more news."

"Thank you," Moyra repeated. "Thank you for letting me know." Both women hung up the phone and sat thinking about the other.

"Well, was that *her*? What was she like?" Linda had only caught one end of the conversation but from the tone of Allison's voice knew that it had indeed been *her* and that something had changed, softened, and opened in Allison.

"Yes," replied Allison, "I'm sure it was her. She sounded, . . . nice. I'm glad," she paused, "we phoned her. Who next?"

⁂

Moyra thought back, not forward, beyond this ending she had known was coming.

They had met at the wedding of her goddaughter Caroline and his nephew Christopher in Florence. Two hundred guests had made the trip to Florence for the long weekend. The wedding had been an extravagant affair. His nephew had spent a university summer internship program at the Villa La Pietra, one of the old Medici palaces. The villa was situated five kilometers outside of Florence, high up on fifty-two acres of grounds which now housed four new villas apart from the original old one. The villa had been poured from the hands of Italian merchants into those of the Anglo-American nouveau-riche community of the nineteenth and twentieth centuries. It became an Englishman's folly as he gathered up the remains of a Medici family's downfall. When the English family money faded along with the antiquities within the villa, a single son had deftly handed the whole estate over to an American university that had been happy to add the pile of bricks, mortar, and olive trees to its portfolio.

Moyra had always been fond of her goddaughter Caroline. She had calmed her friend Jenny's fears when Caroline had found a way to move through her time at university taking a year in New York, and Moyra had given her blessing and encouragement for the final summer session at this villa.

As a young woman Moyra had missed out on a European tour and was always uneasy in the arrogant assurance of Mediterranean beauty. The history of Italy, its ancient heritage, its art, had never caught her. She did not understand the paintings, she did not see the dreams of their churches reaching to their God. But on this weekend in early June, the cool comfort of the Villa La Pietra protected her from the intense heat of the sun and soothed her. Slowly she began to appreciate the high and low thick hedges that shielded the walkways through the terraced gardens surrounding the villa and gave way to the olive groves below. On the evening before the wedding she had discovered the lavender beds. The tiny blossoms were just beginning to swell and the green stalks turn mauve. The bed was alive with movement. Moyra bent down further to look more closely at the bees and butterflies, both still working in the evening light and warmth. She counted at least four different kinds of bees and even more of butterflies. The butterflies she recognized from her own childhood but there were also little winged creatures flitting from blossom to blossom, looking like hummingbirds. She bent down again, peering at them more closely. The more she looked the more of them she saw, there, there and then even more over there. Their brown wings moved so fast that only flashes of orange and white could be seen as they darted and hovered from flower stem head to head. A long beak seemed to probe the flower heads and they moved like noisy miniature spaceships plucking nourishment. She was completely absorbed in her searching and did not notice the man who came up the steps from a garden below and now stood behind and beside her.

"That is the Death Hawk moth but it has a prettier name, The Lavender moth."

"Oh." She turned and looked up at the man who was standing quietly and smiling gently at her. She felt herself become very weak. "Oh," she said again, "that is a pretty name. I like that. They look like hummingbirds."

"They do, don't they? But actually they are moths and are found all over this part of Tuscany and even, I believe, in Southern France. As moths, they feed mostly in the evenings and are very prolific, as you can see." There was a pause as they both looked down at the lavender bed moving not from the evening breeze that was stilled in this part of the garden but from the bees, butterflies, and moths that were working the bed as fast as any farmer harvesting his summer hay before an approaching storm.

"Hummingbirds are from South America," he added, wanting to say something more.

"Yes, that was what was confusing me. They are beautiful though, aren't they?"

"Yes. I love this part of the garden. It is my favorite place here, among," he glanced up at the towering villa now looking rather stern in the evening light, and gestured to the grounds above them, "all of this."

Moyra stood up and the man moved a half step so that he was beside her. In silence they looked back at the bed, busy with factory intent and a beauty beyond humanity. The evening bells of the Duomo began to ring, building steadily with the Christian call to prayer that was followed in the city by the souls moving within the cloistered walls of the cathedral. He looked at the woman beside him. Her body relaxed in soft curves. She was dressed with a slightly too-young casualness for what he suspected was her age. But her summer chinos looked travel-comfortable and the slightly oddly cut top that draped across her chest was intriguing rather than distasteful. Old open-toed sandals showed a pair of pretty feet with well-manicured toenails. Her curly brown hair was pinned up but still tumbled down around her face. She wore no wedding ring.

"Are you here for the wedding?" he asked.

"Yes," she smiled back at him. "I should be getting ready for this evening's reception I suppose, but I just wanted to have a look around first."

"Me too. Have you been here before?"

"No. Never. This is a lovely spot though, isn't it?" With that tight phrase she dismissed any further appreciation of all that Florence might elicit.

"It is a lovely spot. My favorite. I always come here first, just to check in. My name's Derrick, Derrick Bradshaw. My nephew is getting married tomorrow."

"Goodness," Moyra smiled at him, "your nephew is marrying my goddaughter, Caroline. I'm Moyra, Moyra O'Sullivan."

"We will be almost related then, tomorrow." He didn't know why he said it, but as he did he smiled at her. "Are you here with family?" he continued.

"No. I'm alone. Jenny, Caroline's mother, was my best friend at school. Is your family with you?"

His words were measured as he replied. "My daughters, Linda and Allison, are here but my wife—doesn't travel much these days." There was an easy silence between them that allowed the other to take in the information given and received. Moyra smiled again.

"I think I had better be going in. I need to change before the reception. Do you know where that is exactly?"

"Yes, go out through the main door and head over to your left. It is around the side. Actually you can see where they are still setting things up."

"Oh right, that's lovely." Moyra turned to leave the lavender, letting her hands run through the flower heads as if in a goodbye. Derrick found himself falling in step with her and just held himself back from letting his hand follow hers through the lavender.

At the reception, Derrick sought out Moyra and introduced her to his two daughters who had accompanied him to the wedding. They were with their husbands and young children who were preoccupying them as they all settled in. They spoke a little at the reception before Moyra was taken away by Jenny to meet more guests.

"Interesting people darling. That one is a bit stuffy. Has a wife at home who alternately drowns and subdues her sorrows in sherry or valium. Though with him as a husband and the girls well married not too sure what sorrows she has. But then, you never know, do you? Maybe he is batting away from home, but I doubt it. Come on, meet Harry and Ingrid, they've flown in from Boston. Can you believe it? The excuses people will make to take a trip to Florence." The rest of the evening was spent in animated cocktail conversation for Moyra as Jenny led her from one group to another, holding onto her friend tightly as she watched this weekend, which had nearly driven her insane with details, begin to flower into the wedding she had always wished for her daughter Caroline. Caroline was happy too. Happy to see her parents happy, happy to see her godmother, and happiest of all that her beloved Christopher was by her side and willing to share this fairyland beginning of their new lives together.

The day of the wedding began with sightseeing for the guests while the bridal party moved through the rituals of preparation. The sun rose and suffused the gardens in heat and light. By 4 p.m. the heat of the hot summer day had been swept away by the gentlest afternoon breezes. As the day waned, the sunlight gave way to candlelight and the bridal party gathered in the formal gardens. The lilies and roses that had been artfully placed in the huge urns beside the marble statues now released their perfume into the still, evening air. Caroline exuded a radiant beauty. Moyra wondered what was it that made a woman at this moment in time glow as if a beacon of fecundity? Maybe that was it, thought Moyra, that a bride carries the hope of birth and renewal for us all. It is she who reaps the seed that is sown within her. At the reception and dinner the speeches were given, champagne was drunk and the younger friends of Caroline and Christopher took over the party. Parents and young children stayed on late into the night, bedtimes long forgotten. The mothers' feet tapping to the music, their husbands taking them to dance a turn or two in remembrance of the romance of their own beginnings. Moyra smiled as she watched. It was at times like these that she felt most alone. Sometimes the husband of a friend would take Moyra onto the dance floor and give her a turn, and sometimes, when they did, she felt their smugness, that she might slip closer into their arms, but that had long ago ceased to be true. Quietly she got up from the table and said goodnight to the last couple sitting there. She could not remember their names and they barely looked up as the man said, "You're off then?"

"Yes. Goodnight. Enjoy the music."

"Oh, we will, we will." And the man started drumming his fingers on the crumb-covered, wine-stained white linen as if reinforcing his enjoyment. Moyra glanced around and saw Derrick talking with one of his sons-in-law. She waved and he must have been watching for her movements as he looked up and waved back. He tried to rise up from his seat and the earnest conversation his son-in-law was continuing. As Moyra left her table, she stepped towards a side path that led her back to the lavender bed. She wanted just one more moment with which to hold the sweetness of a memory a little closer to her. Suddenly Derrick was by her side.

"Are you leaving?"

"Yes. I have an early start tomorrow. Just wanted to say goodnight to the bees and those moths you showed me before I left."

"I'll come with you. May I?"

"I'd love that." She smiled up to him and down to herself, recognizing that this short stroll would become part of this weekend's memories. They reached the lavender and stood together enjoying the other life that gave it movement, released its sweet perfume, and that had no care for their watching.

"You go back tomorrow?"

"Yes. And you?"

"I will stay a day. Do a little sightseeing with the grandchildren. Then go home on Tuesday. It's been wonderful to meet you. I'm wondering, I'd like to ask you, could we meet up for a drink in town? Would you mind that?" He didn't quite know what he was saying or how he was saying it. All Derrick was aware of was that here was comfort, sweetness, and light laughter. He was as drawn to Moyra as the bees and moths were to the nectar hidden in the lavender. He wanted to bury his head and body into this flower and be encased in its sweet perfume.

"Yes. That would be lovely. I'd love that. Let me give you my number. The machine is always on if I am at work." Derrick took out his little green engagement diary and opened it to the day of the wedding. As Moyra spoke he carefully wrote her name, Moyra O'Sullivan, and phone number.

020 7483-3847.

That was how it had all begun. Five years ago, thought Moyra. It has been a wonderful five years.

⚜

Allison put the phone down and turned to Linda.

"Well?" said Linda.

"Well—I think we've met her, years ago at Christopher's wedding. Do you remember, she was talking with father at the reception, and then I saw them together at supper, after the wedding. She is quite a high-powered research doctor or something like that."

"Do you really think we have met her?

"I do. What was that date again?" Alison turned back to the desk and pulled forward the old diaries from five years ago.

"Look. Here it is. Why didn't I see that? Friday, June twelfth, fly to Florence. Remember? We spent the week there. Father couldn't leave mother for that long. He flew in on Friday, the wedding was on Saturday and he stayed an extra day to take the children sightseeing. Mother was still upset at him for leaving her when we got home. Don't you remember that week?"

"Yes, yes I do," replied Linda, then she laughed. "Sebastian got heat stroke or Cathedral stroke and we all suffered along with him." The sisters laughed together, then paused before getting serious once more.

"Come on, best get going then," said Linda and Allison reached for the phone. They began by calling Uncle Jimmy. By four-thirty they were done and had phoned in the notice for *The Times* and *The Telegraph*. They got up, stretching, from their seats in the study. Linda went downstairs to the kitchen and put the kettle on while Allison went to wake Elizabeth for tea.

Elizabeth lay in the center of her double bed. Hers for a few years now since Derrick had taken himself off to his dressing room. He said it was because he didn't want to disturb her with his late night reading but in truth it was her sleeping body, made brittle and dry from alcohol, that he had long withdrawn from as firmly as he had reached for her once fresh, yielding flesh. Elizabeth had tired of him early in their marriage, taking refuge first in gin and tonics before dinner and then adding wine at lunch and valium for her remaining nerves through the day. It was a deadly mix but one that had not yet killed her. She would submerge deeply into sleep, her mouth wide open, snores ebbing and flowing from her throat until she woke in a befuddled daze in the morning. This afternoon she lay curled in the center of the bed. Her skirt was folded neatly on the chair and her slip lay taut over her bloated tummy. Her legs, encased in good hose, were still trim, for apart from her liver-extended belly, Elizabeth looked a well preserved woman for her age of seventy-two.

Allison stuck her head around her mother's bedroom door and then tiptoed down to the kitchen.

"Let's take a tray up to her room. She's still sleeping and must be tired."

"What do you think? One of us should stay with her. We can't just leave her tonight."

"I'll stay. You go home. I'll stay through the service." Allison couldn't bring herself to say funeral. "We'll figure out what to do after that." The kettle boiled and Linda made the tea. She put three pieces of Dundee cake, her father's favorite, on a plate and tore three sections of paper towel off to serve as a paper napkin. Her mother hated crumbs on the bed.

Moyra waited a day after reading the words in *The Telegraph*. She arrived at Buckingham's before ten-thirty in the morning. Moyra wanted to see for herself that death had claimed him. The young mortician on duty asked her to wait while they brought Mr. Bradshaw out.

Derrick lay lightly in his coffin. His dark suit was pinned back behind him so that it looked softly fitted as if the slightness of his flesh was also the normalness of his body. His mouth was shut, his nostrils pinched and eyelids closed as if in a tense sleep. His eyebrows, which had always been unruly, growing like moths' antennae looking for light and which had become wilder during the last few months, were now clipped and gave his face the look of a prone mannequin. It was his trim eyebrows that startled Moyra more than any other aspect of his appearance.

Moyra pulled the chair that was against the wall closer to the coffin and sat down. She reached over the coffin brim and covered his cold clasped waxed hands with hers. She stroked him slowly, leaning forward, looking into the face that she had so often covered in warm and hot kisses and had loved to feel the heat of its returning gaze. She stroked his chest over the white shirt and under the club tie. Her hand glided down his body, stumbling over the hard nub of the insertion tube that had drained out his body's fluid and filled him with embalming liquid. It traveled down his leg feeling the shin bone sharp against her hand. His feet stuck up, encased in his best shiny black shoes. A mistake, she thought. He had always worn brown, even with this dark suit. Moyra became calm, looking at Derrick and stroking his body. She leaned against the coffin's edge, smiling with her eyes full of tears into the face that no longer looked at her and the body that no longer stirred with that look. Slowly she became aware of voices, of a man and a woman outside in the waiting room. Moyra sat up, unsure what to do. Discreetly the young mortician knocked on the panel behind the curtain and came into the room, "Excuse me madam. Some of the deceased's family are here. Would you like them to come in, or," smoothly "maybe you would like to come this way?"

"Yes. Yes, of course. I don't want to disturb anyone. Let me come with you." Moyra got up from the chair and with a final smile said goodbye to the unseeing face of Derrick. She turned and followed the young man out of the room, along a short corridor to another exit door. She smiled again as she watched him move the curtain covering the upper glass panes of the door to be sure that no relatives lingered in the parking lot. They must be used to this, she thought wryly and shook her head.

Moyra arrived early on Tuesday morning and waited outside the church. She had dressed smartly but with a little smile, wearing her laciest black underwear. Her shoes were flirtatious rather than sensible for the March cold morning. She had wrapped a blue and white silk band from a summer dress around her black hat in remembrance of how on a summer afternoon Derrick had unwound the same sash from her waist before taking her all ways onto his lap. She longed for a cigarette, something she had given up on meeting Derrick but now the craving almost propelled her into asking a stranger for a light. Nervousness, not the cold wind, made her tremble. The night before, after she had dictated her final laboratory reports, she told her assistant not to expect her at the hospital today. She would not look at another slide, not see what the cells showed for the unknown name on the slide, not write a report, that with its knowledge would release or doom a family to the path she had just trodden. She was doing them a favor, *you don't need to know, don't want to know, just yet*. For once there is knowing there is no unknowing. Denial and ignorance are sometimes better. *Trust me, I know.* All these thoughts she had repeated in her mind as she dressed that morning. Now she was here, at the church, the morning air was cold and she felt chilled as she waited outside around the corner of Saint Mark's Church on the Marylebone Road.

She watched the mourning family preceding Derrick's hearse file out of the church and enter their black cars to follow the hearse to a cemetery. She watched as another hearse brought Derrick's body to the steps and parked in exactly the same spot in front of the church. She watched as three black limousines pulled up behind the hearse and the doors were opened. She watched as Derrick's sons-in-law helped Elizabeth out of the first limousine and their wives gathered the grandchildren around them to walk up the steps as a family. Moyra looked at Elizabeth, encased in her black suit, a big brimmed hat and short pert veil.

The church steps became crowded. There were now more people going up and into the church than coming down out of the tall, old, wood church doors. Moyra joined them, following behind Uncle Jimmy, his wife Angela, and their grandson Sebastian. People were nodding hello to one another. Sometimes words were spoken but mostly the voices were hushed.

Moyra kept her head down. She chose a pew at the back of the church and sat in a discreet, secretarial manner. From the far back corner she could watch Derrick's friends and colleagues as they filed into the church to pay their last respects. She recognized no one. They had never minded or missed mingled company. The organ played softly, keeping everyone soothed and calm. It wasn't until after the service when the crowd of mourners blocked the exit from the church that voices were raised in recognition and confusion. The family had been led back into the side waiting room from where they would normally follow the hearse out to the cemetery, but Derrick had not been clear about his last wishes and Elizabeth remained vague. Later there would be a cremation and his ashes returned to the family.

The crowd made its way slowly down the church steps. A reception was to take place at the city club where Derrick had spent less time than his family supposed. Linda and Allison's husbands mingled with the guests, urging and encouraging them to go onto the club for a drink and "a spot of lunch."

"Won't be much, just some sandwiches and such." Linda and Allison remained with their mother in the waiting room. Allison looked back out at the crowd of people and saw a woman standing alone. She pinched Linda.

"Look. I think that is her. Moyra. I think I recognize her. Shall I say something?"

"Yes, do. I think you are right. Yes, say hello, see if she wants to come on to the club." Allison went outside of the waiting room and edged between the dark-suited friends of her father's.

"Excuse me, sorry, just want to get by. Thank you so much." She finally reached Moyra's side. Moyra looked over at her, her mouth open, not sure whether to be afraid or to smile. Allison smiled.

"Excuse me. Are you Moyra O'Sullivan?"

"Yes. Yes, I am." Her voice fell from the question.

"I'm Allison. His daughter, eldest," she added, not yet able to say Derrick to this woman she did not know.

"I think we've met before. At my cousin's wedding, in Florence. Where you met—my father." Now it was Allison's voice that faded away. Moyra came to her rescue.

"Yes. That is where Derrick and I met." The relationship was now acknowledged.

"Your cousin married my godson. Yes, we [an inclusive we] met there." Moyra turned to Allison now, one woman to another, lover and daughter, and continued, "How are you doing? How is your sister," she hesitated, "your family?" Moyra reached out her hand and in the manner of a woman already wearing this loss among her others touched Allison's arm. Allison did not recoil but stood silently accepting this gift.

"We're tired," she answered truthfully, "very tired. The last few weeks were," another pause as she tried to find a word that would not give Moyra more pain, "tiring." She finished lamely and then added, "It wasn't just Daddy."

Moyra broke in, "Yes. I know. The whole family, it must have been very hard. I'm so sorry." And the sorrow and loss that they both felt flowed from the heart and hand of each through the arm to the hand and heart of the other.

"Please come," said Allison. "Please come back to the club. I do want to talk with you more. So does my sister, Linda. It will be all right, I promise. Just for a few minutes." Suddenly Moyra felt a wave of protective love from and for this woman whom she barely knew but who had been known and loved by the man who loved her. They were not too distant in age, Moyra maybe ten years the daughter's senior, the age of a good aunt.

"Yes, all right. I'll come just for a few minutes to say hello to your sister, if you are sure it will be all right."

"Oh good. Yes. That would be so nice. You know where it is?" Allison replied quickly.

"Yes. I know," and they both smiled knowing that there was more knowing than not knowing about them both. Allison took Moyra's hand and squeezed it as they said goodbye for the moment.

Moyra walked down the church steps and across the entrance to the Marylebone High Street where it was easy to find a taxi that had just discharged its passengers to the scrubbed and geranium-box-bordered steps of a Harley Street clinic or a boutique on the now fashionable high street. A taxi stopped quickly. Moyra got in and gave the address. With a tight u-turn the driver faced his vehicle into the city and St. James. Moyra sat back, looking out at this London. The sun came out briefly, making her think of the way Derrick would look at her when they had taken such a taxi in the city together for an evening event. Her lips tightened, holding back the tears that she had not yet shed. There was only memory now. The taxi swung down the discreet street off of St. James and came to a stop outside the Doric pillars holding up the balcony over the central doors to Derrick's club. She had often come here with him. In the early days when they both believed that they were just friends. And then, later, as acknowledged lovers. Moyra paid the driver and got out.

The doorman bowed to her and offered an impassive, "Good afternoon madam." He guided her to the reception room, filled with the black-suited men and women from the church. Moyra bypassed the queue of people clustered around a table holding a book of condolence to sign. She reached for the glass of champagne offered to her by a young waitress that, with relief, she did not recognize.

"Thank you," she said as she looked at the young woman and wondered who took these club jobs now. She stood pausing for a moment, sipping the champagne before wandering the perimeter of the room, visiting the old portraits hanging on the wall. She had strolled here before, waiting for Derrick or lingering after he had left. The faces in the paintings stared back down at her. Often she had felt a compassionate welcome from these men dressed in the colonial military uniforms of the previous century and the turbaned and tuniced officers who had been so very reluctant to return home. She did not have long to wait before Allison arrived with Linda. For many minutes Allison was caught up speaking with this uncle and that junior partner. Finally she excused herself and found her way to Moyra's side.

"I'm so glad you are here. Sorry that I'm so late. Mother wasn't very well and so I have sent her home."

"Shouldn't you be with her?"

"No. It's all right. Our daily lady, Sarah, is with her. She will be fine and sleep for the afternoon. May I introduce you?" Before Moyra could reply Derrick's two sons-in-law were by her side. Martin and Ian were both middle-aged men who had held their bodies in moderate check and wore their dark suits well. Allison and Linda had shared their secret discovery of Moyra with their husbands who were both now eager to meet her. Having lived through their years with Elizabeth, they were glad for the old boy that he had found happiness. It was Martin who brought up the indelicate question.

"Anyone decided what we are going to do with him?" Martin did not speak unkindly, he just wanted things done. A still silence fell in the circle on the carpet that they all stood around.

"No dear," said Allison, used, as they all were, to these outbursts from Martin. "No. We've not decided, have we Linda?" She asked this last question wearily. It was a topic that held no comfort to the sisters. They had no help from their mother and they didn't know what Derrick really had wanted. Where his soul would rest most easy in death.

"Do you have any ideas?" Moyra asked the question softly to the women.

"No. Not really. We're looking for somewhere—somewhere he really loved. Maybe the sea. Maybe we should cast him out to sea." A pause and then Allison turned to Moyra, "Do you have any?"

"Oh. No, I don't think so," and another pause before she added quietly. "But he often talked about the lavender beds at the Palazzo, where your cousin was married." She just caught herself from saying, where we met, but all three of the women were thinking that. "He found them so alive. Do you remember, the butterflies and the moths and the little birds. All so beautiful and so peaceful."

"That's right," said Allison. "He did love that time away. Maybe we should think about it. Florence. We could take another trip. What do you say?" She turned with a smile to her sister who was looking sad again.

"Well, maybe. It's something to think about anyway."

"Good. That's settled then." Martin took another gulp of wine and snagged a smoked salmon sandwich from the waitress as she went past with the tray.

"What do you do then? I've heard you are a doctor?"

"A pathologist," Moyra replied. "I don't see patients, just slides." And she gave a little laugh, happy with this turn in the conversation which at another time she would have found rude but now eased her away from the focus of Derrick's bodily remains. Martin cocked an eyebrow, not letting her deflect her work so easily.

"Any particular specialty?"

"Not really. I work for a teaching hospital and so much comes through there. All sorts really. And you?" She firmly turned the questions back onto Martin, already knowing he could not refuse her.

"Gastrologist, up in Leeds. Surgery. You know, the usual thing." He too shrugged his life's work away, and it was Moyra's turn to face him and draw him back towards her, and the reason they were gathered together.

"These last few weeks must have been hard for you, with your wife—Allison—spending her time down here." A silence could have laid between them but Martin responded quickly.

"Yes—and no. We knew it was coming of course, the last couple of years. And the girls were devoted you know, just devoted to their father. This is what they had wanted to do, right from when they knew he was ill. And he was very grateful. So it was fine really. And the end was short."

"Were you able to help at all?" Moyra asked in a manner of politeness rather than curiosity but still his answer shook her.

"Oh no. Good Lord, no. Wouldn't want to interfere down here. Gerald Bruner, he's an excellent man. It would not have done at all. Couldn't have that. You know how it is, understand, I'm sure."

"Yes, yes. I see." Moyra spoke quietly, taking in the fact that for this man of technical precision and science how things seemed was more important than how things were. Moyra had also been stopped short in her efforts. Derrick had been clear with her from when he first learnt of his illness and understood the journey now before him.

"You mustn't get involved my dear. No trying those back doors or telephone connections. You mustn't expose your concern. It will be all right." And so she had followed his wishes even as they both had known it would not be all right.

As Moyra looked at Martin her brief anger at him left her as quickly as it had arrived and she simply smiled.

"It is time I was going." She turned to look for Allison and Linda and say her goodbyes to them also. They did not urge Moyra to stay longer, recognizing her rhythms and needs.

"Please, let us stay in touch," Allison asked.

"Yes, of course. You have my number."

"Let me walk you to the door."

"No need. I'll be fine."

"It's no trouble. I need to step out of here for a moment." Allison smiled at her and the two women walked together out of the reception room and through the foyer. Allison reached for Moyra's hand to hold once more.

"Goodbye then, and thank you. Take good care of yourself."

Moyra returned the pressure of Allison's hand. "Goodbye. You take care of yourself too, and your family. Thank you for your kindness to me." Moyra turned and passed through the door held open again by the liveried footman. Carefully she walked down the steps to the street, holding herself upright.

As Allison watched Moyra reach the street, she saw the loneliness of solitude fall and settle onto her shoulders and lead her away.

Epilogue: A True Story

AS THEY WANDER ALONG the bank of Rome's Tiber River, Hanna pulls her extendable leash to its full length. Her head is down and her terrier nose twitchingly alert as she smells out the secrets of the cobblestones that pave the wide river walkway. Over the years flotsam garbage has met and sealed together, locking into clumps of debris that cling to the river banks. Ducks fertilize and bring seed to the growing mounds. Fireweed, grasses, and brambles sprout and occasional shrubs try to stand upright, taller than their roots can go deep.

It is high summer. Hanna and Daphne have come to Rome for six weeks. Without Hanna as her constant companion, Daphne would be desolate. Her husband, James, leaves early in the morning for work and returns late in the night. She holds in her body the early middle-age wisps of autumnal beauty. She knows very few words of Italian and is intimidated by the haughtiness of the waiters who themselves are but claiming their place in the universe.

Three times a day the dog and the woman walk the city. In the Villa Borghese Hanna romps, happily darting in and out of the shrubbery, sniffing out the squirrels and birds that live in the gardens. She goes expectantly with Daphne to the Campo dei Fiori market where they shop at the stalls for juicy, ripe pears, cured salamis, and perfect cheese.

But the river walk is different. The speed, width, and dark depth of the water as the river channels deep through the length of the city is dangerous. Sometimes Daphne or Hanna will see the rats, bigger than any land rat, a primeval ancestor to the Ratty of *The Wind in the Willows*. Daphne holds tight to Hanna's leash as they walk along, back up the steps and across the Ponte Sisto Bridge to the center of the city.

They walk through the Campo Marzio courtyard in front of Italo Calvino's home, along the smaller alleyways where, only at night, young children are seated in front of the looms holding heavy tapestry rugs in need of repair. The children are dark skinned. The girls have light cotton frocks that don't cover their knees. They sit cross-legged, hunched over the tapestry, lit and yet shaded by a single light bulb centered on their work.

It is late afternoon when they return to the Piazza San Lorenzo and time for another cup of coffee. Daphne chooses a table and Hanna resignedly sits down beside her. The waiter comes over and Daphne orders. "Un caffe latte, per favore," she says softly before she lowers her head shyly and turns back to face the empty coffee table.

Two tables away sits another woman, maybe ten years older than Daphne, on the other side of middle age. She is holding tightly to a leash. On the end of her leash is a small Yorkshire terrier.

The two dogs notice each other at the same time. From the safety of their mistress's chairs and bound by the leashes that hold them close they stare at each other. The young Yorkshire terrier is dressed in a tartan harness and leash with a matching bow in her forelock. She is excited, curious, and hopeful. She barks first. 'Yap, yap,' she goes. Hanna raises her head and barks a single, mature reply.

Daphne snaps the leash, gently, as an apparent reprimand. She raises her eyes, searching for the reason of Hanna's barking and sees the cheerful little terrier face under her owner's chair. She smiles at the little dog who wiggles at the stranger's recognition. Hanna sits up and looks cross. The older woman takes another sip of her coffee.

"Bongiorno Signora, mi scusi. Do you speak English?" Daphne asks, knowing instinctively that she does.

"Yes. I speak English." The two women sit looking at each other across their tables at the cafe in the Piazza San Lorenzo. The dogs are quiet now, hopeful that their job is finished. They both sit down beside their respective chairs and wait. They know better than the curious sparrows that there will be no crumbs falling from these tables.

"Do *you* speak any Italian?" the older woman asks as if questioning a college school applicant.

"Solo un po. I'm English."

The older woman sniffs. The English, she thinks, most of them as bad with language as the Americans but worse in their attitude of expecting their Englishness to be a reasonable excuse for their laziness.

"I have been learning Italian in the park, walking with my dog. It has been fun but limited to *'Come si chiama, lei? Quanti anni ha? E sembra maschile o femminile?'*" She laughs and draws from the older woman a small smile in return. Daphne takes a deep breath and continues. She does not get to speak to many people outside of the park or the market and knows this could be her only chance for a real conversation that is not bound to her existence.

"Could you tell me, are there any choral concerts playing in Rome at the moment?" She asks for choral concerts, they seem safe, classical and yet not too deep. She can barely distinguish Handel from Bach or Beethoven but she enjoys some classical music. Choral music brings her back to the chapels of her childhood and might even, in a Catholic country, bring her some comfort from her solitude.

The older woman tilts her head back as if to sniff again, but does not.

"The choral season is over now. Do you like music?"

Daphne nods.

"Yes," but she thinks she should own up to her lack of education. "But I don't know very much about it." The older woman softens, sensing the younger woman's vulnerability and loneliness. Her own stretches out before her, running parallel to the remaining days of her life, shining like a long, twisted, black branch that is stripped of interesting foliage. She changes the subject and asks, "Do you like dogs?"

"Oh yes. I do." Daphne's face brightens. She smiles and reaches down to pat and scratch Hanna on the head. As she speaks Hanna looks up expectantly and then warily, watching the other dog.

"I don't," says the older woman abruptly. She absentmindedly jerks her little dog's lead even though the dog is sitting perfectly still while keeping her eyes on Hanna.

"I bought this for my husband. He named her Trixie. But it was too late. My husband died. Now I have to care for her." There is a long silence as the two women take in the words.

Finally Daphne responds, "I'm so sorry. But Trixie looks so sweet. My dog's name is Hanna. I would be quite lost without her. My name is Daphne, Daphne Blanford." The older woman nods at this introduction and replies, "I am Bianca, Bianca Leonardi." Together they take a sip of their coffee. There is another, longer silence as they each roll the other's name around in their mouths, savoring the new words. Bianca speaks first, resuming the connection.

"What are you doing in Rome?"

"My husband is an art director. He is working on a film at Cinecittà. We are here for six weeks before going on to Paris." Bianca shifts her posture slightly, sitting more upright in her chair.

"I was a painter when I first met my husband." She takes in a deep breath before continuing with her most powerful statement, "My husband was Puccini's nephew."

Daphne's reaction is all that Bianca could have wished for. Her eyes widen and she smiles in acknowledgment. Among all the museums and relics of the ancient past Daphne had walked through and around nothing compared to this moment. She knows she is in the presence of a living touchstone of art in history.

"Oh," is all she can say. But it is the right oh and Bianca relaxes and settles into the telling of her story. Both dogs relax too, understanding the engagement of their respective mistresses. They each extend their heads onto their front paws and half-doze under the chairs on the piazza. They sigh in unison and wait.

"I was a young painter when I met my husband. He was much older than me. I continued to paint throughout our affair and even after, when we finally were married. When Puccini was in Rome he would come to the house. My house first and then, when we were married, my husband's house, where I live now. When Puccini traveled he would always write to my husband. Apart from his wife and son my husband was his only relative and they stayed in touch. I have all of his correspondence."

"Oh. How wonderful. Have you always lived in Rome?"

"And Paris. I lived in Paris as a young woman. I came to Rome after I met my husband, to be with him and then we lived here." Bianca paused, a hyphen in her thoughts as she comes to the last few years of her story.

"My husband was so much older than me but it was I who became ill first. Last year I returned to Paris for heart surgery. The best heart surgeons are there and I knew them. Besides I did not want to bother my husband with the surgery. He would only worry and fuss. He was too old. But there were complications, you know, with the surgery, an infection, and I nearly died." She lets out a sigh that settles on all the complications the heart has to suffer and then continued.

"My husband became worried and then upset that I was away so long. In the autumn he came to Paris, discharged me from the hospital and brought me home to recover. I did. He saved my life. But I was still so afraid that I would die and so worried for him to be lonely that I bought him this dog." Bianca raises her left hand from the table, pulling on Trixie's leash and lifting the dog's head for a moment. Trixie opens her eyes in surprise.

"But it was too late," Bianca resumes. "My husband he was so old, so frail. He could not care for me, it made him ill, and he died. I recovered and now all I have is this dog." She pauses for a moment. "And it is I who am lonely."

The two women sit in silence once more. The story lies gently between them like a soft fog floating over the two semi-bare coffee tables in front of them.

"I'm so sorry," Daphne says quietly, for the second time in this conversation. "Loneliness is hard." She pauses again before continuing, "How good it is that you have Trixie. She looks so sweet. She must be a dear companion."

"It is nothing." Bianca replies, her thin lips set in a line. "I am still lonely. But she makes me walk which I must do to become stronger. It is a long process." Bianca sighs and then lifts her chin and glances off to her left. For the first time Daphne notices the man standing a few feet away, at attention, behind Bianca. He is a small, trim, middle-aged man contained in a cardigan. His hair is an applied, shiny, black color, and he seems younger than Bianca, though that is not necessarily so.

"You are here Raymondo?"

"Si Signora." With a small bow Raymondo moves forward to claim Trixie's lead and stand close behind Bianca's seat expectantly, waiting for her to rise and leave. But she does not. She reaches into her large bag and from its depths brings out a faded cream card. Only then does she rise out of her chair, suddenly urgent and passionate, and thrusts the card towards Daphne.

"This is my address. Take down my phone number," she orders. "You must come to tea. I live on the top of the steps, next door to Valentino's. We . . ." she looked brightly at Trixie for the first time that afternoon,

". . . after lunch we walk down together and then two hours later he," she tips her head back, "drives down to pick us up. Have you got my phone number? Call me." She says the last sentence in a rush of feminine longing and conspiracy.

Daphne pulls a pad and pen from her bag and begins to write the number from the faded card placed on the table.

Nursing Notes for
The Bell Lap

Nursing notes, written about and for the patient, are not the same as doctor's orders. Even when doctors have the time, in teaching rounds or conferences, to elicit and share their patients' stories they are different from the listening nurses' notes. Though many of our observations may overlap, this is a primary, separate skill from that of the physician. For nurses are honed to receive our patients' pain, fear, and loneliness, and it is in that receiving that we can hear and heal.

I think for nurse-writers the struggle is quieter—as many things are—than that of the modern-day physician-writer, though no less determined. In whose footsteps do we follow? Who lights the candle so that we may tread safely, even firmly, through illness, life, and into literature? It was my nursing tutor, Sister Boisher, who handed me the slim *Medicine in Its Human Setting*. It is a book I love, and has stayed close by my side, traveling from home to home since 1962. And so, for me, story has stayed the vehicle with which to share my gifts.

My last student rotation before final exams was in Accident and Emergency, A & E, as it is also known. Rushing on duty, late, I bumped into a gurney parked in the entranceway. A diminutive elderly lady was strapped firmly in place. Had she had a fall, a nasty turn? I can't remember. But I do remember standing beside her while her eyes searched mine as I tried to reassure her. She looked at my stripes and, recognizing I was a third year student, asked how soon were my finals. "Then you are ready for your buckle, Nurse? Are your parents giving you one?" I confessed that I didn't think the idea had crossed my mother's mind!

"I'm going to give you mine," she said firmly. For she too was a nurse. I thought no more about it until two weeks later I found a small package in the nurses' mailbox addressed to me. In it, wrapped in crumbled tissue paper, was a silver buckle from my nurse-patient. I never knew her story, but dimly (for I was young) I did realize that she had one, and that, with her gift, I was being handed a sacred trust. What was this promise that I have held my life long? It took me many years of living and nursing before I could understand and articulate it. For whatever else we do with our lives—beyond the ward, the surgical suite, and our communities—for those of us for whom training as a nurse comes in our formative years, it molds who we are and we never really stop nursing.

Now—in my own Bell Lap—this book is my silver buckle for you.

What are the thoughts, wrapped in my writing, that I can share with you?

Susan Sontag said,

> To me, literature is a calling, even a kind of salvation. It connects me with an enterprise that is over 2,000 years old. What do we have from the past? Art and thought. That's what lasts. That's what continues to feed people and give them an idea of something better...[1]

So what are the reasons for you to read this little book?

Or, in "school-speak," what are the key issues and learning points you can reflect on and take with you after reading these stories?

Will these stories help you pass physiology or chemistry or cardiac arrhythmia exams? Doubtful.

But they will help you be a finer nurse or physician.

In the hurry of tending to the overwhelming desk-work and heavy machines that need watching as much as the person they are attached to, here is a moment to see, through story, that your patients are people with their own lives and stories that come before your care.

Here is Sontag again:

> Illness is the night-side of life, a more onerous citizenship. Everyone who is born holds dual citizenship, in the kingdom of the well and in the kingdom of the sick. Although we all prefer to use only the good passport, sooner or later each of us is obliged, at least for a spell, to identify ourselves as citizens of that other place.[2]

In *The Bell Lap* we can see that, whatever our social-economic status, illness comes to us all, from Tony, the prominent neurosurgeon in *A Drop of Blood*, to Jennifer watching from her perch in the pedicure chair in *It Says Love*.

In *It Says Love*, how much illness is there and who is ill? Is it Jennifer with her loneliness and benign neglect, from herself and her daughter, or the young woman with her possibly/probably abusive boyfriend?

Mr. Tims' Morning is a reflection back into a place and time. It is an example of how, with less, we could give our patients more of what they needed.

> Compassion is an unstable emotion. It needs to be translated into action, or it withers.[3]

How can you show that now?

What have we nurses lost from our toolkit?

For one: the ward kitchen, where a really good hot cup of tea can come from. I do pray that this exists somewhere still!

Another is the truly hot washcloth.

I'm sure you can think of other places where casual intimacy has been made more difficult.

That casual intimacy is a big, open door to understanding and empathy.

Here is a question—an exercise if you will—to learn one personal or familial fact from every patient, or their family, given directly to you and added to your nurses' notes. Think of it, one fact from every nurse, shared among you all.

In *The Brigadier, His Buggy and the Butterfly* we see an independent, yet rigid, spirit immersed in a natural fear and forced courage.

Can we, as do the doctors in this story, recognize the Brigadier's fear along with that of his wife? Can we see where each tried to protect the other?

How to acknowledge that?

Morning Coffee. Apart from severe status epilepticus or tonic–clonic seizures (which used to be called grand mal), and emergencies or neurological testing, when do nurses see fits or seizures?

With the additional increase of street drug and alcohol use and self-medication comes judgment. Do you pre-judge this disorder?

What stigma and fear does epilepsy still carry for the nursing, medical, and general population?

> It is not suffering as such that is most deeply feared but suffering that degrades.[4]

Betty in *The Museum Visit* and Gwendolyn, in *Spring Fever*, have their own agendas.

These ladies come from different social backgrounds and different degrees of optimal wellness. How they manage to carry them out speaks of the will and the life force in each of us.

Who helps them and in what ways? Who recognizes their spirit, their need to be the self?

Who is willing to risk helping them in this safety-oriented world?

How will you, as nurses in similar or more confined settings, help these women maintain their individuality and independence?

Phone Calls and *The Waiting Room* speak to the onset or recognition of disease. Both stories are at a beginning, leaving us knowing there is more to come for the patient and their families. Where will you as nurses fit in? Can you look back and imagine what their lives were/are before they came to your care?

What will happen in their lives when they and/or their families leave you?

How much should you wonder and wander along these thoughts?

How far is far enough, or too far?

The questions raised in *The Vigil* stand alone for me.

I have seen, and continue to see, the doctor in *The Vigil* over the years. Here is a physician for whom disease and the fixing of are the challenges and rewards of his calling. For the Doctor Goughs of the world, death is still an unacceptable outcome, one they cannot bear to be a part of, or certainly engage in.

Do they "miss" the deathbed in an unconscious but determined manner? Is it that once death becomes inevitable, they walk away?

And then I wondered what would happen if they were caught, trapped by the bedside of a beloved. Would love, loyalty, and decency enable the good doctor to stay and be vigil to the end?

The role of the volunteer fire department speaks also of a community.

In both rural and urban environments there is a comradeship between the men and women who are the nurses, paramedics, and fire fighters. This companionship can help ease a patient's transition from one place, home and familiar, to the next, the hospital and unknown.

In *Doctor Patel Comes to Tea* Mrs. Andrews never actually sees a registered nurse. Her care comes from her daughter and her doctors. In this story, maybe more than the others, you will find awareness leading to fear. The fear of what is to come. How will this all end for her? Parts of that unfold in the following two stories, *The Visitor* and *The Dentist*.

There is a very good analysis of *Doctor Patel Comes to Tea* by Arthur Frank in *Stories of Illness and Healing: Women Write their Bodies*.[5]

The Letter M and the *Epilogue* can also be taken as a loose pair.

Earlier this year a report came out of Brigham Young University stating that

Loneliness and social isolation are just as much a threat to longevity as obesity.[6]

This ancient universal truth helps account for the modern obsession that we hold to e-mail, Facebook, Twitter and Instagram. These are all ways of staying connected within a real or virtual community that sometimes feels far away and out of reach.

These stories speak of loss and loneliness for those families, loved ones, and friends left behind. These ladies will also become your patients. They too have their stories, their memories, and their characters. Do not discard them.

The themes of *The Bell Lap* include:

How do we care and how do we show we care?

Watching a loved one at the beginning and through to the end of the paths of illness.

Where are the nurses? Are they at a bridge point, a crossing-over, in the middle?

Nurses are teachers of patient care: to the patients, to their families and at times to young doctors.

What do you want? The question posed by Atul Gawande in *Being Mortal*.[7]

Nurses can and do ask this question too.

What are the nursing skills that these stories can enhance in you?

The power of observation.

Receiving and listening to your patients.

Learning to anticipate needs.

How far to go? Where to intervene with families, physicians, and loved ones of good intent.

Nursing is not a passive activity. We can guide, act, and speak up when we see a patient's well-being compromised.

Can you reflect on what was, what is, and what is to become of nursing care?

References

1. Garis L. Susan Sontag finds romance. Interview, *The New York Times*. 1992 Aug 2. Reproduced with permission.
2. Sontag S. *Illness As Metaphor*. New York: Farrar, Straus and Giroux; 1978. p. 3. Reproduced with permission.
3. Sontag S. *AIDS and Its Metaphors*. New York: Farrar, Straus and Giroux; 1989. p. 125. Reproduced with permission.
4. Sontag S. *Regarding the Pain of Others*. New York: Farrar, Straus and Giroux; 2003. p. 101. Reproduced with permission.
5. Frank A. The negative privilege of women's illness narratives. In: DasGupta S, Hurst M, editors. *Stories of Illness and Healing: Women write their bodies*. Ohio: Kent State University Press; 2007.
6. Holt-Lunstad J, Smith TB, Baker M, Harris T, Stephenson D. Loneliness and social isolation as risk factors for mortality: a meta-analytic review. *Perspect Psychol Sci*. 2015; **10**(2): 227.
7. Gawande A. *Being Mortal: Medicine and what matters in the end*. New York: Metropolitan Books/Henry Holt and Co; 2014.

Index

Alexander the Great, 121
arthritis, 13, 23, 72, 100

Beal, Tony, 7–11
Bell Lap, use of term, 2–3
Betty, 41–52, 148

Chanel, Coco, 46, 48, 50
Christmas, 29, 99–104, 118–19
compassion, 1, 147

dementia, 89–98
dentures, 107–14
disease, recognition of, 148
Doctor Patel, 89–98, 149
Doctor Riley, 3–5
dogs, 139–43
'dying floor,' 54

epilepsy, 148

fear
    awareness leading to, 149
    of inevitable death, 81, 86–7, 148
    nurses receiving, 145
    of rejection, 53
    and stigma, 148
fire fighters, 83–6, 148–9
funerals, 115–37

'Good King Wenceslas,' 29
Graham, 1–2, 4–5
Gwendolyn, 53–60, 148

heart attack, 53, 77
heart surgery, 14–15, 17–20,
    142–3

hip fractures, 53–4
hospice, 117–18

intimacy, casual, 147

Jennifer, 33–8, 147

Lisa, 61–2, 64–9
loneliness, 141, 143, 147, 149
    nurses receiving, 145
    of patients, 28
    and secret intimacy, 105, 119, 137

military men, 13–25, 107
Mr. Tims, 27–32, 147

nightmares, 19, 23
nursing homes, 97
nursing notes, 145–50

paramedics, 83–4, 149

radiotherapy, 28

seizures, 39–40, 82, 147
self-medication, 126, 129, 147
social isolation, 149
Sontag, Susan, 146
stroke, 44, 83–8
student nurses, 4, 28, 56, 145–6
surgery, waiting for, 71–9

test results, 66–9

volunteers, 29, 73, 83, 148–9

wellness, optimal, 148

About the Author

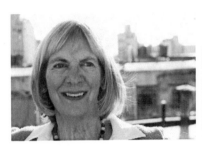

Muriel A. Murch was born and grew up in England, graduating as a nurse in 1964. In 1965 she married Walter Murch in New York City and they motorcycled to Los Angeles, California, relocating to the Bay Area in 1969.

Muriel added a Bachelor of Science in Nursing from San Francisco State University in 1991 whence came *Journey in the Middle of the Road: One Woman's Journey through a Mid-Life Education*, published by Sybil Press in 1995.

Her short stories and poetry are included in several university press anthologies and on-line journals focused on the writings of nurses and women's health. Among them are *Between the Heart Beats: Poetry and Prose by Nurses* (1995) and *Intensive Care: More Poetry and Prose by Nurses* (2003), both published by Iowa University Press. *Stories of Illness and Healing: Women Write Their Bodies* was published by Kent State University Press in 2007. *The Story of Christmas: The Muscovy Duck* was published in a limited edition in 2010.

Muriel continues to write stories and poetry while occasionally producing independent radio programs for KWMR.org at 90.5, 89.9, and 92.3 FM.

She and her husband divide their time between London and their grown family.

www.murielmurch.com

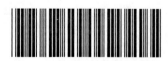